CONTINUOUS PERIPHERAL NERVE BLOCK TECHNIQUES

An Illustrated Guide

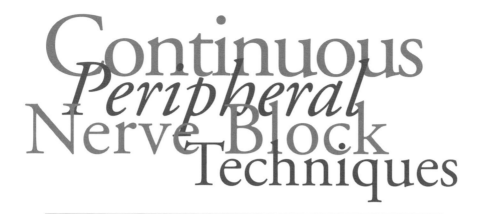

Continuous Peripheral Nerve Block Techniques

An Illustrated Guide

Jacques E. Chelly

*Professor, Director of Clinical Research and
Orthopaedic Anesthesia and Orthopaedic Acute Pain
Department of Anesthesiology
Houston, Texas, USA*

Andrea Casati

*Department of Anesthesiology and Intensive Care
San Raffaele Hospital
Milan, Italy*

Guido Fanelli

*Department of Anesthesiology and Intensive Care
San Raffaele Hospital
Milan, Italy*

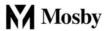 **Mosby**

EDINBURGH • LONDON • NEW YORK • OXFORD • PHILADELPHIA • ST LOUIS • SYDNEY • TORONTO • 2001

MOSBY
An imprint of Elsevier Limited

ISBN 0 7234 3270 8
First published 2001
   Reprinted 2002, 2003, 2004

British Library Cataloguing in Publication Data
A catalogue records for this book are available from the US Library of Congress and the British Library.

Note
Medical knowledge is constantly changing. As new information becomes available, changes in treatment, procedures, equipment and the use of drugs become necessary. The editors, authors, contributors and the publishers have taken care to ensure that the information given in this text is accurate and up-to-date. However, readers are strongly advised to confirm that the information, especially with regard to drug usage, complies with the latest legislation and standards of practice.

your source for books,
journals and multimedia
in the health sciences
www.elsevierhealth.com

The
publisher's
policy is to use
**paper manufactured
from sustainable forests**

Printed in China
C/04

Commissioning Editor: Daniela Famigli
Project Manager: Susanna Garofalo
Copy Editor: John Ormiston
Design and Illustration: Studio Sismondo-Rome
Index: Louise Bleazard

CONTENTS

SECTION 1   INTRODUCTION AND GENERAL CONCEPTS   1

1   HISTORY   3

2   GENERAL CONCEPTS AND INDICATIONS   11

3   COMPLICATIONS   21

SECTION 2   EQUIPMENT AND DRUGS   27

4   LOCAL ANESTHETICS   29

5   EQUIPMENT   37

Contents

Contributors

FERDINANDO ALEMANNO, MD

Professor of Anesthesiology
University of Verona
Verona, Italy

PIA DI BENEDETTO, MD

Department of Anesthesiology and Intensive Care
Orthopedic Trauma Hospital
Rome, Italy

LAURA BERTINI, MD

Department of Anesthesiology and Intensive Care
Orthopedic Trauma Hospital
Rome, Italy

FRANCESCA KAYSER ENNEKING, MD

Associate Professor of Anesthesiology
Department of Anesthesiology
College of Medicine
University of Florida
Gainesville, Florida, USA

BRIAN M. ILFELD, MD

Fellow Regional Anesthesia
Department of Anesthesiology
College of Medicine
University of Florida
Gainesville, Florida, USA

MARIA MATUSZCZAK, MD

Visiting Associate Professor
Department of Anesthesiology
Medical School
University of Texas
Houston, Texas, USA

Acknowledgments

We gratefully acknowledge the contribution of the following, who have provide slides, radiographs or other illustrative material:
Carola Achilli, Elisa Cerchierini, Domenico Nucera, Lorenzo Quario, Mara Scandroglio, Angela Sciascia.

FOREWORD

Regional anesthesia has made great strides in the past several decades. New techniques and new research have improved the performance and documented the superiority of regional blockade. Regional techniques have been identified as superior for outpatient surgical anesthesia and postoperative analgesia. Inpatient epidural infusions have been clearly identified as the superior modality of analgesia following thoracic and upper abdominal surgery. Opioid and/or local anesthetic infusions have become the mainstay of postoperative pain management for the inpatient surgical population. Their documented advantages include not only pain relief, but also a reduction of the cardiac and respiratory morbidity associated with the perioperative period and to facilitate patient discharge. Peripheral regional techniques have also been shown to improve recovery and rehabilitation after orthopedic surgery, and thus are receiving increased interest and utilization.

There is a price to pay, however, with neuraxial analgesia. Motor blockade and sympathetic blockade are infrequent but still present, and they limit the use of these techniques in some patients. Although more effective than systemic opioids, neuraxial opioids still carry the risk of pruritus, nausea, and rare respiratory depression. These limitations make the neuraxial techniques inappropriate for outpatient analgesia, which is unfortunate since outpatient surgery now constitutes the majority of cases in North America and an increasing proportion of the European surgical experience. The use of peripheral nerve blocks, on the other hand, provides an isolated targeted analgesic regimen that can provide the same degree of analgesia without the drawbacks of epidural infusions or the side effects of systemic opioids. Peripheral nerve blocks are especially suited to the outpatient population, for which ambulation and position are usually not limited. Analgesia can be prolonged without the side effects of nausea and drowsiness associated with systemic medication. There are many reports of successful prolonged analgesia with the long-acting local anesthetic agents available to us today, especially in the lower extremity where block duration is longer. Still, single injection techniques are limited to the maximum duration of the local anesthetics, and rarely exceed 24 hours. Patients experience pain for longer periods than this, and the side effects and rehabilitation are often limited by inadequate analgesia. Oral opioid analgesics are effective, but not without their side effects. In the ideal world, we could provide our patients with the benefits of peripheral nerve blockade for an indefinite period until their surgery had completely healed and their rehabilitation was complete. We may not be able to achieve this goal, but the use of continuous peripheral nerve blocks described in this text can take us a long way down this desirable path.

As the authors identify in the opening chapters, continuous peripheral blocks have been performed in the past, and have been quite effective. Until recently, the techniques were cumbersome because of limitations in the equipment that was available. In the past several years we have seen the introduction of a number of needle and catheter developments that greatly facilitate the placement of continuous peripheral nerve catheters, as described in Section Two of this text. We have also witnessed the introduction of drug delivery systems suitable for long-term peripheral nerve infusions. We now have both the disposable simple elastomeric balloon pumps and the sophisticated power-driven infusion devices for use in hospitals, or even at home in a portable model. The drugs available now also have a better safety margin, especially if we are concerned about rising blood levels with long-term infusions. We have discovered additives, such as clonidine, that can enhance our analgesia while simultaneously reducing the local anesthetic dosage requirement. The combination of all these developments has fostered the production of this textbook.

This text is an overview of the development of continuous techniques as well as an in-depth manual for their performance. It provides an excellent description of the techniques involved in both the upper and lower extremities, as well as the approach to wound infiltration and pediatric applications. The illustrations and explanations here can improve not only the performance of basic blocks, but also can greatly facilitate the learning experience for the practitioner who wishes to move up to the level of continuous infusions.

There is no doubt a greater technical challenge in the placement and maintenance of a catheter for postoperative analgesia. The time commitment is greater and more attention to detail is required for insertion, securing and maintenance of the catheters, and provision of the appropriate infusions. Nevertheless, it is clear that this is the way of the future. This is a modality that will provide the alternative to epidural opioid infusions for inpatients for peripheral surgery. It has already been shown to be extremely effective and even superior to epidural opioids for lower extremity orthopedic procedures. It is also the technique that holds the most promise for continued analgesia in the outpatient setting. The use of the techniques described in this book will give all anesthesiology providers an opportunity to step forward into this new millennium with a wider range of tools to improve their service to their patients and surgeons. This is clearly the next step for anesthesiologists, and this book is a most welcome and important stepping stone to all of us in this regard.

Michael F. Mulroy M.D.

Department of Anesthesiology
Virginia Mason Medical Center
Seattle, USA

PREFACE

The management and care of patients during the perioperative period has become a focal point of great interest to different specialists, and in this the new generation of anesthesiologists will play a crucial role in perioperative medicine, including pain treatment. Relevant progress has been made in the past few years in our understanding of the mechanisms and pathways involved in the modulations of pain, as well as in the development of new therapeutic tools to provide satisfactory pain relief after surgery. Simultaneously, also because of the development of new and safer drugs and equipment, peripheral nerve blocks for pain treatment have enjoyed a considerable resurgence of interest in both Europe and the USA.

Peripheral nerve blocks are very effective for intraoperative anesthesia and postoperative pain control in orthopedic patients, and are also associated with less morbidity than central nerve blocks. However, their duration, which does not exceed 14–18 hours even with long-acting anesthetic solutions, limits their effectiveness for postoperative analgesia, since most of the in- and outpatient orthopedic procedures for upper and lower extremities require postoperative pain control for more than 24 hours. For this reason, continuous perineural infusion techniques are increasingly being used to prolong the analgesic effect of peripheral nerve blocks after surgery in orthopedic patients.

A number of studies support the usefulness and clinical relevance of continuous peripheral nerve blocks. These not only show the positive effects on the efficacy of acute pain treatment, but also show important benefits in immediate functional outcome and the reductions in both serious postoperative complications and hospital length of stay for the patient after surgery. For these reasons the interest in continuous perineural infusion techniques is growing rapidly, and continuous peripheral nerve blocks will replace both single-shot nerve blocks and continuous epidural analgesia in many orthopedic patients.

In our departments the use of continuous perineural infusion techniques has greatly expanded in the past few years with highly successful results. However, although landmarks and techniques do not substantially differ between single-shot and continuous nerve blocks, special skills are required when using a continuous perineural infusion, not only for catheter placement, but also for postoperative follow up. This last point is actually crucial, especially as to be effective continuous perineural infusion techniques must be part of a multidisciplinary and multimodal approach to postoperative pain management, according to the new philosophy of perioperative medicine. For this reason, all specialists (including surgeons, anesthesiologists, recovery and ward nurses, physical therapists, and pharmacists) who take care of patients must coordinate their effort to improve the well-being and the final outcome of the patient throughout the perioperative period. Finally, serious consideration must to be given to which needles, catheters, and equipment are required to optimize success and safety.

Our commitment in writing this book is to provide the clinician with the philosophical background behind continuous peripheral nerve blocks, along with practical descriptive anatomic landmarks and tips for performing continuous peripheral nerve blocks for surgery and postoperative pain relief. It is our hope that use of this illustrated guide may improve the clinician's skills as well as patient care, and still address the economic issues of today's healthcare environment.

Jacques E. Chelly, MD, PhD, MBA
Andrea Casati, MD
Guido Fanelli, MD

1

INTRODUCTION AND GENERAL CONCEPTS

HISTORY

J.E. Chelly

Continuous peripheral nerve blocks: upper limb

In 1946, Paul Ansbro described the placement of a supraclavicular catheter to block the brachial plexus and enable the injection of procaine 1% to prolong the duration of anesthesia in patients undergoing surgery of the upper extremities. Especially interesting is that the apparatus used to infuse the anesthetic solution consisted of a 10 ml Luer lock syringe and a two-way valve similar to that used in the Hingson–Edwards continuous caudal method. The technique was based on the use of a blunt needle placed to the lateral side of the subclavian artery in contact with the upper surface of the first rib after obtaining paresthesia in the upper limb. Then the needle was secured to the patient's skin by inserting it through a cork before block placement. Adhesive strapping over the cork prevented the outward displacement of the needle while it was held securely in the cork *(Figure 1.1)*. Ansbro used injections of local anesthetics, starting with 40 ml and a total volume of 120 ml for 1.5 hours up to 220 ml for 4 hours of surgery. This article is remarkable from several standpoints:

- first, the author recognized the need for negative blood aspiration before injecting the local anesthetic solution;
- second, he described the indications for supraclavicular block, which remarkably correspond to the present indications for this approach;
- third, the reported side effects were surprisingly minor (pallor

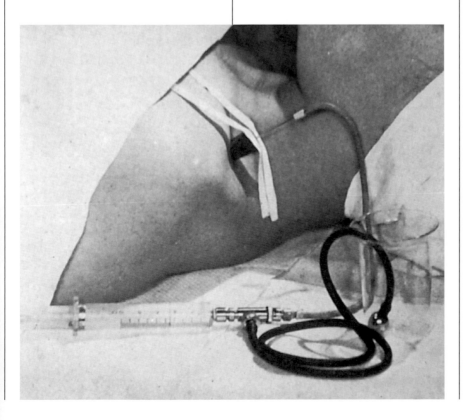

Technique described by Ansbro in 1946 to place a supraclavicular catheter: the needle is held in place using a cork fixed to the skin with drapes, while a system of tubes allowed unidirectional injection of the anesthetic solution. (Reproduced from Ansbro 1946, with permission from Elsevier Science.)

◀ **Figure 1.1**

and sweating in only three patients); and

- finally, Ansbro presented the concept of preferential sensory block by using a 1% concentration of procaine with good sensory block, instead of a 2% concentration of procaine, which produced sensory and motor blocks.

In 1951 Sarnoff and Sarnoff described the use of a catheter placed in proximity to the phrenic nerve with an 18-gauge introducer needle. After the appropriate placement of the introducer needle, a 12.5 cm polyethylene catheter *(Figure 1.2A)* with a contained stylet was introduced in proximity to the phrenic nerve *(Figure 1.2B)*. The introducer needle was withdrawn along with the stylet before a 23-gauge needle was inserted in the open end of the tubing. Of spe-cial interest in this article is the first mention of the use of a nerve stim-ulator and the application of an electric current to the stylet to obtain a diaphragmatic motor response to verify the proper place-ment of the catheter *(Figure 1.3)*. The catheter was maintained in place for several days, and during this time it was injected with local anesthetic solutions to treat intractable hiccups.

For the next 34 years, continuous perineural infusion techniques were developed and their indica-tions extended, but initially the focus was on upper extremity blocks, specifically the brachial plexus. In 1969, De Krey et al. reported the use of the interscalene approach with a 'Rochester'-type plastic needle. The authors used 15- to 18-gauge needles and a tan-gential approach to the brachial plexus. After eliciting a paresthesia, the needle was advanced by at least another 0.5 cm before withdrawing the stylet and advancing the plastic portion of the needle by another 1 cm. The authors used this tech-nique in 25 patients and main-tained the catheter for several days, not only for anesthesia but also for postoperative analgesia with repeated injections of local anes-thetics in volumes and concentra-tion similar to those used for single injections.

In 1977, Selander published a study of 137 patients in whom an axillary catheter was placed for hand surgery. The catheter was a 47 mm long Teflon cannula for intravenous use with a hollow stainless steel stylet. It was intro-duced to rest tangentially at the side of the artery inside the brachial plexus sheath. The block

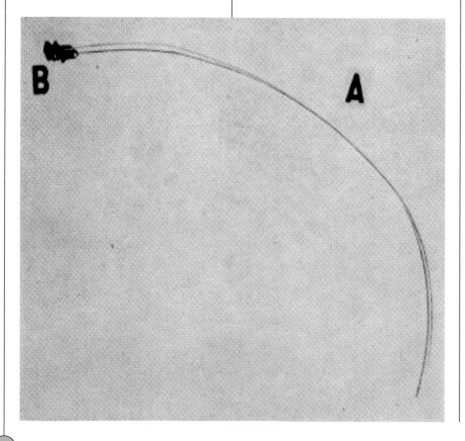

A. Polyethylene catheter.
B. Metallic stylet contained inside the catheter.
(Adapted from Sarnoff and Sarnoff 1951, with permission from Lippincott, Williams & Wilkins.)

◀ **Figure 1.2**

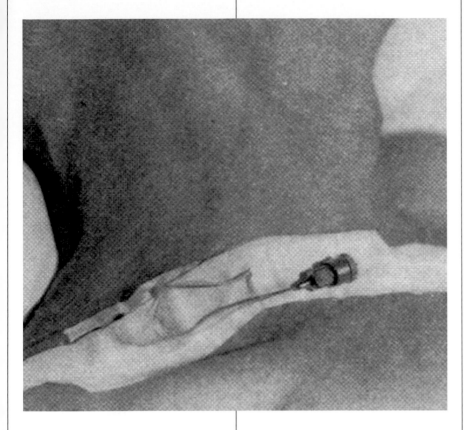

Figure 1.3

Phrenic catheter placed by Sarnoff and Sarnoff (1951) to treat a resistant hiccup. (Reproduced from Sarnoff and Sarnoff 1951, with permission from Lippincott, Williams & Wilkins.)

was achieved with an injection of 30 ml to 50 ml of mepivacaine. The catheter was removed after surgery. Failure occurred in 5.1% of cases. Complications of this approach included vascular puncture in 24% and accidental paresthesia in 39% of cases.

In 1978, Manriquez and Pallares reported on the placement of an interscalene catheter for repeated 20 ml injections of bupivacaine 0.25% every 6 hours to prolong the sympathetic block and pain control for 4 days in three patients. In 1982, Matsuda et al. reported the use of 50 continuous supraclavicular or axillary catheters for postoperative pain management in patients undergoing upper extremity reimplantation. An intravenous polyethylene catheter with a 16-gauge 30 mm metal needle was used for the supraclavicular approach, along with a paresthesia

technique. A 19-gauge 50 mm flexible Teflon needle with a 23-gauge hollow metal stylet was used for the axillary approach, along with a paresthesia technique. The supraclavicular catheters were infused with either lidocaine (lignocaine) 1% with epinephrine (adrenaline) or a mixture of bupivacaine 0.5% and lidocaine 1%. When using lidocaine 1% with epinephrine, the authors initially injected 30 ml followed by intermittent injections of 15 ml (1.5–2.7 h), while when using a mixture of bupivacaine 0.5% and lidocaine 1%, the authors initially injected 40 ml followed by intermittent injections of 20 ml (1.2–4.3 h). They reported a 94% success rate with one pneumothorax in the supraclavicular group. In 1983, Sada et al. reported the use of continuous axillary infusions of mepivacaine 1.5% for anesthesia in

597 patients undergoing reimplantation of fingers. They had a failure rate of only 3.7%, 2.8% with systemic toxicity, 0.5% nerve injuries, and one hematoma. A 23-gauge 50 mm intravenous Teflon catheter was introduced where the pulsation of the brachial artery could no longer be felt under the pectoralis major muscle, with the catheter pointing toward the apex. The authors searched for a paresthesia, which they believed to be better than the 'click' in determining that the tip of the catheter was within the perivascular sheath. In 1984, Ang et al. described a new approach for the placement of an axillary catheter that increased the rate of success and decreased the rate of vascular puncture. The arm was abducted at 75° and externally rotated with the forearm flexed at the elbow. The point of insertion was 40 mm below the axilla, medi-

al to both the biceps muscle and the median nerve. A 50 mm long 19-gauge needle was inserted at an angle of 20° to the skin. A flexible guide was introduced into the lumen of the needle and advanced 100–150 mm until a resistance was felt. The needle was removed and an 18-gauge catheter inserted into the introducer plastic catheter.

Tuominen et al. (1987, 1989) seem to have been the first to report the use of continuous interscalene infusion with bupivacaine 0.25% at a rate of 0.25 mg/kg/h for 24 hours for the postoperative pain management after shoulder surgery. Although this technique was more effective than a single injection of 1.25 mg/kg of bupivacaine 0.5%, it was also associated with local anesthetic accumulation (plasma levels increased from 0.7 µg/ml to 1.1 µg/ml) and clinical symptoms related to local anesthetic accumulation, such as dizziness and confusion.

Haasio et al. (1990) studied the effects of an interscalene injection of bupivacaine 0.75% (20–28 ml) followed by a continuous infusion of bupivacaine 0.25% at a rate of 0.25 mg/kg/h. Next, the effects of an interscalene continuous technique on ventilatory function were investigated by Pere et al. (1992, 1993). Patients first received an interscalene injection of bupivacaine 0.75% with epinephrine (20–28 ml) followed by an infusion of bupivacaine 0.25% or 0.125 % (plus fentanyl) at a rate of 5–9 ml/h for shoulder surgery. In these experimental conditions, Pere et al. demonstrated an ipsilateral hemidiaphragm paresis. Borgeat et al. (1997) introduced, for the same indications, the use of patient-controlled interscalene continuous

infusion of bupivacaine 0.15% with a basal rate of 5 ml/h, a bolus of 3–4 ml, and a lockout period of 20 minutes. This technique proved to be safe and effective, without the previously reported clinical symptoms of toxicity, and it was superior to the use of patient-controlled analgesia (PCA) morphine.

In 1998, Iskandar et al. reported the use of continuous axillary infusions of either 0.1 ml/kg/h of bupivacaine 0.25% or 0.1 ml/kg boluses of the same solution with a lockout period of 1 hour for postoperative analgesia after severe hand trauma. They demonstrated that the patient-controlled approach was associated with less bupivacaine consumption, and better pain control and patient satisfaction. In 1999, Singelyn et al. demonstrated that interscalene basal infusion of 5 ml/h plus boluses of 2.5 ml with a 30 minute lockout period produced similar pain relief benefits to those of 10 ml/h continuous infusions in patients undergoing open shoulder surgery. These approaches provided better pain relief than interscalene patient-controlled injections of 5 ml boluses with a lockout period of 30 minutes. The use of the patient-controlled interscalene analgesia technique was also associated with a significant reduction in local anesthetic consumption, and therefore was the recommended technique. Similar results have also been reported by Borgeat et al. (2000), who evaluated the effects of interscalene infusion of ropivacaine 0.2% at a rate of 5 ml/h plus a bolus of 3 or 4 ml with a lockout period of 20 minutes for 48 hours. In this report, the authors demonstrated that this technique did not significantly affect ventilatory

function, and provided better postoperative analgesia than the continuous intravenous infusions of 0.5 mg/h nicomorphine. In 2001, the same group demonstrated that the use of patient-controlled continuous interscalene infusion of 0.2% produced selective sensory block in patients undergoing major shoulder surgery. They compared the effects of ropivacaine 0.2% and bupivacaine 0.15% (to account for the difference in potency between ropivacaine and bupivacaine) infused via an interscalene catheter on the sensory and motor function after major open shoulder surgery. The study design included a patient-controlled method with a basal rate of 5 ml/h plus a bolus of 4 ml with a lockout period of 20 minutes for a total volume of 17 ml. The infusion was preceded 6 hours earlier by the injection of an initial volume of 40 ml of ropivacaine 0.6% or bupivacaine 0.5%. Hand motor function was evaluated using handgrip strength. With this study design, Borgeat et al. (2001) clearly demonstrated that bupivacaine and ropivacaine provide similar postoperative pain control, but ropivacaine 0.2% better preserved motor function. This study provides the strongest clinical evidence that ropivacaine is more suitable than bupivacaine for the continuous perineural infusion of local anesthetic in the management of postoperative pain for orthopedics, because of the preferential sensory block that ropivacaine produces at that concentration. Indeed, in most cases the preferential sensory block is required for the functional recovery of orthopedic patients as it allows immediate postoperative physical therapy.

Continuous peripheral nerve blocks: lower limb

Probably because of the extensive use of spinal and epidural techniques for lower extremity anesthesia and analgesia, it was only in 1978 that Brands and Callanan reported the first lumbar plexus placement of an epidural catheter using an 18-gauge 150 mm spinal needle. The technique was used for preoperative and postoperative analgesia in 21 patients with a fractured neck of the femur. The lumbar plexus catheter allowed discontinuous injection of 15 ml of bupivacaine 0.5% with epinephrine and provided 4–6 hours of analgesia. They reported that a continuous lumbar plexus block allowed the use of opioids to be minimized and provided pain relief at rest as well as during mobilization. The landmarks used were similar to those proposed later by Parkinson et al. (1989) and are recognized to frequently result in epidural placement of the catheter; interestingly, systolic blood pressure dropped in all patients with successful block.

In 1984, Smith et al. reported the use of a continuous sciatic block for ischemic pain of the toes and foot in a 77-year-old diabetic patient. This sciatic catheter was placed using a posterior approach and a 16-gauge cannula with a metal trocar connected to a nerve stimulator. The catheter was introduced 6 cm and infused with bupivacaine 0.5% at a rate of 3.0 ml/h for 48 hours.

Dahl et al. (1988) demonstrated that the continuous femoral infusion of bupivacaine 0.25% at a rate of 0.35 mg/kg/h for 16 hours reduced the postoperative morphine requirement and pain score in patients undergoing open knee surgery. The bupivacaine plasma concentrations associated with these infusions were around 1 μg/ml and below the toxic level (4 μg/ml). Using a similar design, Anker-Moller et al. (1990), using a double-blind design, demonstrated that bupivacaine 0.125% produced a similar postoperative morphine sparing and pain relief than bupivacaine 0.25% in patients undergoing open knee surgery. In 1990, Ben-David et al. published the case of a 71-year-old who received a continuous psoas block for surgical repair of a hip fracture. In 1992, Edwards and Wright confirmed the data previously obtained that the continuous femoral infusion of bupivacaine 0.125% at 6 ml/h provided satisfactory postoperative pain relief after a total knee replacement.

In 1992, Vaghadia et al. reported the use of continuous lumbosacral blocks for anesthesia in elderly patients undergoing lower extremity procedures (knee arthroscopy, above the knee amputation, debridement of the right thigh, and harvesting of skin graft). The placement of the catheter was achieved using a 17-gauge Tuohy needle and enabled the injection of contrast solution to confirm the spread of the local anesthetic mixture. In 1996, Mansour and Bennetts demonstrated that a single sciatic block using a parasacral approach combined with a continuous femoral infusion of bupivacaine 0.125% and fentanyl 2 μg/ml at rate of 10 ml/h and a bolus of 10 ml of the same solution every 4 hours *pro re nata* for 28 hours provided appropriate post-operative analgesia in patients who underwent major knee surgery, either anterior cruciate ligament (ACL) or total knee replacement. During the same year, Spansberg et al. reported the value of a continuous lumbar plexus block of bupivacaine 0.25% at a rate of 0.14 mg/kg/h preceded by a bolus of bupivacaine 0.5% at a dose of 0.4 mg/kg for postoperative pain control after a femoral neck fracture. However, the continuous lumbar plexus was combined with acetylsalicylic acid administration.

Singelyn et al. (1997) described an original continuous popliteal sciatic technique for postoperative analgesia after foot surgery. With a 60 mm 18-gauge plastic catheter mounted on a metallic introducer connected to a nerve stimulator, they used the Seldinger technique. After the injection of a bolus, the catheter was infused with bupivacaine 0.125% with sufentanil 0.1 μg/ml and clonidine 1 μg/ml at a rate of 7 ml/h for 48 hours. Patients also received 1 g proparacetamol intravenously (i.v.) and 10–20 mg intramuscular piritramide *pro re nata*. Singelyn et al. (1997) reported technical problems in 25% of patients and that in 10% the infusions had to be stopped prematurely.

In the same year, Morris and Lang (1997) reported the placement of a parasacral perineural catheter to enable a continuous block of the parasacral plexus, and particularly the sciatic nerve, in two patients who underwent an ankle arthrodesis and below-knee amputation, respectively. Using a 17-gauge insulated Tuohy needle, the authors placed an 18-gauge epidural catheter in a parasacral position. The catheter was used for anesthesia and acute postoperative analgesia of the sciatic nerve. It was infused postoperatively with bupivacaine 0.1% at a rate of 8 ml/h for 48 hours. In 1998, Singelyn et al. compared the effects of continuous femoral infusions to PCA morphine and epidural analgesia for the management of acute postoperative pain in patients who underwent total knee replacement. They demonstrated that continuous femoral infusions of a mixture of bupivacaine 0.25%, sufentanil, and clonidine at a rate of 10 ml/h for 48 hours resulted in a 60% reduction in postoperative morphine consumption and a better immediate functional recovery (as indicated by a greater range of passive motion using a continuous passive motion machine). In addition, the use of the perineural technique was associated with a 20% reduction in the immediate postoperative period and initial rehabilitation period. According to the study design, each patient also received proparacetamol 1 g q8h.

Using an iliofascial 'double-pop' technique, Ganapathy et al. (1999) studied the effects of continuous femoral infusions of bupivacaine 0.1% and 0.2% versus saline at a rate of 10 ml/h for 48 hours for acute postoperative pain in patients undergoing total knee replacement. They demonstrated that bupivacaine 0.2% provided better postoperative analgesia than either bupivacaine 0.1% or saline. Ganapathy et al. (1999) advanced the catheter 15–20 cm cranially and reported that only 40% were located superior to the upper-third of the sacroiliac joint in the psoas sheath (ideal location). Although the use of continuous infusions of bupivacaine 0.2% and 0.1% result-

ed in a decrease in postoperative morphine requirement versus that of saline, Ganapathy et al. also reported that within the bupivacaine groups, the patients with catheters in the 'ideal location' required even less morphine. This suggests a relationship between the pain-relief effectiveness of the technique and the location of the catheter, especially with low concentrations of bupivacaine. Finally, Ganapathy et al. demonstrated that bupivacaine 0.2% also resulted in a better immediate functional recovery, as indicated by a greater range of motion on the first postoperative day.

In 1999, Chudinov et al. reported the effects of repeated injections of 1–2 mg/kg of bupivacaine 0.25% with epinephrine via a catheter placed in the psoas compartment using an 18-gauge epidural needle and a loss of resistance technique in patients with a hip fracture. The authors found that this technique was appropriate for pre- and postoperative analgesia, but inadequate for anesthesia except in three of the 40 patients studied. In the same study, Chudinov et al. also reported an anatomic evaluation performed in 15 cadavers: they showed that in 10 of the 15 cadavers the catheters were inserted successfully in the psoas compartment and in two cases a bilateral spread was observed.

In 1999, Capdevila et al. studied the effects of continuous femoral infusions of lidocaine 1% with 1 µg/ml clonidine and 0.03 mg/ml morphine at a rate of 10 ml/h for postoperative analgesia and functional rehabilitation in patients who underwent total knee replacement. They confirmed that continuous femoral blocks provided bet-

ter postoperative analgesia, facilitated recovery and functional outcome, and reduced the length of rehabilitation by 30% compared to PCA morphine.

Chelly et al. (2001d) confirmed that continuous femoral infusions of ropivacaine 0.2% for 48 hours in patients undergoing total knee replacement provided better postoperative pain control than epidural analgesia and PCA morphine. They also confirmed that, with this technique, the morphine requirement was greatly reduced and the immediate functional recovery accelerated compared to epidural analgesia and PCA morphine. Furthermore, they reported that the use of continuous femoral infusions was also associated with a 20% reduction in the duration of hospitalization, a 60% reduction in total postoperative blood required, and an 80% reduction in serious complications following surgery.

Singelyn et al. (2001) used a solution of bupivacaine 0.125% plus 0.1 µg/ml sufentanil and 1 µg/ml clonidine and showed that a patient-controlled femoral injection of 5 ml with a lockout period of 30 minutes (total 10 ml/h) was associated with the smallest local anesthetic consumption and the greatest patient satisfaction in patients undergoing hip replacement. In this study, all the patients also received ketorolac 30 mg at the induction of anesthesia and q8h after surgery for 48 hours. More recently, Chelly et al. (2001c) demonstrated that continuous lumbar infusions of ropivacaine 0.2% decreased the postoperative morphine requirement by 60% in patients who underwent open reduction and internal fixation of an acetabular fracture. They also showed that this technique allowed patients to ambulate independently 1 day earlier than those who received PCA morphine for postoperative pain control.

All these data support the usefulness and clinical relevance of this new approach to postoperative pain relief, not only for the positive effects on the efficacy of pain relief, but also for the important benefits in terms of the final outcome for the patient after surgery.

Continuous peripheral nerve blocks: upper and lower limbs for pediatric patients

Very little is known about the use of continuous infusion techniques in children. In 1979, Rosenblatt et al. described the use of an axillary approach in a 15-year-old boy who had amputated his index finger with multiple tendon lacerations. An 18-gauge, 50 mm Teflon-coated intravenous cannula threaded over a 22-gauge 8.75 cm spinal needle was used along with a nerve stimulator. After the catheter had been positioned and 20 ml of a mixture of bupivacaine 0.75% and chloroprocaine 3% injected, the surgery was performed. In the recovery room the position of the catheter was confirmed by injecting 10 ml of Renografin 60; then, bupivacaine 0.25% at 10 ml/h was started and continued for the next 48 hours. This report appears to be the first to describe the use of continuous infusion of local anesthetics with a continuous volumetric infusion pump. Plasma levels indicated that this arbitrary rate of infusion produced a plasma level of bupivacaine below the toxic threshold. In 1980, Rosenblatt first

reported the use of a femoral catheter in a 13-year-old child who underwent surgery for a patella repair of the right knee. Even though initially Rosenblatt had planned an epidural technique, which was converted into a femoral catheter placement after both parents adamantly opposed a 'spinal-like anesthetic'.

In 1994, Fewtrell et al. reported the use of a continuous axillary infusion in an 11-month-old child. They used an 18-gauge insulated needle and a nerve stimulator to locate the axillary sheath. Once located, 3 ml bupivacaine 0.25% in 10 ml saline was injected. Next, a catheter was inserted to 4 cm. Analgesia was maintained with a continuous infusion of bupivacaine and diamorphine (15 ml bupivacaine 0.5% plus 1 mg diamorphine diluted to 50 ml at 2 ml/h). The catheter was maintained for 10 days. In 1994 Johnson published the result of a series of 23 children, average age 9 years (range from 15 months to 14 years), with traumatic femoral fractures treated using a continuous femoral infusion of bupivacaine 0.25% at a rate of 0.3 ml/kg/h. The catheter was inserted prior to surgery and maintained for 2–5 days. In this report a standard 18-gauge epidural kit was used with an iliofascial approach. One child developed a localized infection at the insertion site after 4 days, while leakage from the insertion site was common. In the same year, Tobias reported on four children, average age 10 years, with femoral fractures who received a continuous femoral infusion using a 3 Fr gauge 6 cm single-lumen central venous catheter placed in the femoral sheath and using the Seldinger and 'double-pop' tech-

niques. The catheter was infused with bupivacaine 0.2% at 4–7 ml/h (0.15 ml/kg/h) after an initial bolus of 0.5 ml/kg bupivacaine 0.25% (maximum 20 ml) with epinephrine. Tobias confirmed Johnson's finding. Paut et al. (2001) reported on the use of continuous fascia iliaca infusion for postoperative treatment of pain after femur fracture in 23 children (average age 9.9 years). Recently, Sciard et al. (2001) reported the use of continuous lumbar plexus block in 2- and 4-year old children.

Continuous peripheral nerve blocks: upper and lower limbs for outpatients

The constant search for increased efficiency and earlier discharge times has led to a constant increase in the number of outpatient procedures in orthopedics. However, it is well documented that more than 40% of ambulatory patients experience moderate-to-severe pain within the first 48 hours after ambulatory orthopedic surgery (Rawal et al. 1998). Although different therapeutic approaches have been advocated, none provide reliable pain control, and pain remains a major concern. Most frequently patients are discharged with oral medication that has limited pain-relief effects. Intra-articular injections of narcotic analgesics or local anesthetics have also been used, but these techniques provide only limited and short-lasting pain relief. Although single blocks are very effective for postoperative pain control after orthopedic procedures, their effectiveness is limited by the duration of action of the available solutions of local anesthetics, which usually does not exceed 18–24 hours. To provide better postoperative pain control in an ambulatory environment, continuous perineural infusions of ropivacaine 0.2% have been used for several indications, including rotator cuff (Chelly et al. 2001b) and hand surgery, ACL and patella repair, and major foot surgery.

Chelly et al. (2001a, b) reported their experiences with continuous interscalene, axillary, femoral, and sciatic infusions of ropivacaine 0.2% in patients who underwent various ambulatory orthopedic surgery. This technique provided very effective pain control for up to 48 hours.

At the present time two types of pumps are available:

- first, elastomeric or electronic pumps, which provide only a constant rate of infusion of 2, 5, 10, or more ml/h; and
- second, an electronic PCA pump that provides a basal rate (0–20 ml/h) and a bolus (0–10 ml) with a variable lockout time (0–60 minutes).

CHAPTER
2 GENERAL CONCEPTS AND INDICATIONS

J.E. Chelly

Introduction

In the past few years progress has been made in our understanding of the mechanisms and pathways involved in the modulations of pain, as well as in the development of new therapeutic tools to provide satisfactory pain relief after surgery. For this reason the prevention and treatment of acute pain has become a focal point of great interest to different specialists, including anesthesiologists.

Although the therapeutic principles that apply to acute pain resemble those that apply to chronic pain, the approach often differs. In fact, postoperative pain differs from chronic pain in both its shorter duration and the requirement for immediate relief; these dictate the development of different protocols. Also, a relationship between the intensity of acute postoperative pain and the duration of the patient's recovery and functional outcome is well established. Furthermore, preemptive and preventive analgesia are concepts that apply to acute postoperative pain only. Finally, it is important to recognize the role of acute pain in the development of chronic pain syndrome.

Irrespective of its nature, pain is not an objective, but rather a subjective symptom. In the surgical as well as medical environment, both intrinsic and extrinsic factors affect the individual's pain threshold.

Acute postoperative pain in orthopedic patients

Intrinsic factors

The intrinsic factors include not only the patient's own threshold, but also his or her preoperative medical and psychological condition.

Certainly, old age does not increase pain threshold, and therefore postoperative pain management in the elderly should be similar to that in younger patients (if age is the only variable). Data related to gender are somewhat less clear. It is possible that women have a higher pain threshold than men, but this difference does not justify providing women with pain treatment of lesser potency than that given to men. However, Sarton et al. (2000) demonstrated that, although there is no difference in morphine metabolism related to gender, morphine is more potent with a slower onset and offset in women.

Preoperative medical conditions

It is well established that patients with diabetic neuropathy may have a higher pain threshold. In contrast, the pain threshold is often lower in depressed patients and in those with

an acute emotional distress, such as that associated with trauma. However, prostration (another psychological response to emotional stress) is more often associated with an apparent increase in the pain threshold. The presence of a preoperative chronic pain syndrome is associated with a very low postoperative pain threshold and often represents a therapeutic challenge, since many of these patients develop tolerances to different analgesics, including opioids and/or different therapeutic modalities.

Although the concept of preemptive analgesia is still the object of passionate debate, it is clear that patients in pain prior to surgery have a reduced pain threshold during the postoperative period. In these patients the intensity and nature of the acute postoperative pain also depends on the preoperative control of their pain. For example, patients who undergo above- and/or below-knee amputations may experience less pain, and develop phantom pain syndromes less frequently, if either neuroaxial or peripheral nerve blocks are performed prior to surgery. The same benefit from the preoperative management of pain applies to patients who undergo spinal instrumentation and have been given cyclooxygenase 2 (COX2) inhibitors (such as 50 mg of rofecoxib) preoperatively. This therapeutic approach has been shown to reduce the need for morphine during the first day following surgery by more than 30% (Reuben et al. 2000).

Concomitant preoperative therapy

It is well established that patients who receive either corticosteroids or nonsteroidal anti-inflammatory drugs (NSAIDs) in large doses (such as patients with rheumatoid arthritis), as well as those who consume large doses of opioids preoperatively (such as patients with spinal injury), have a decreased pain threshold. These patients often develop a tolerance and even a dependence on corticosteroids and narcotic analgesics, and only respond to large doses and multiple drugs. Therefore, the acute postoperative pain of these patients must be treated as aggressively as possible. It is only after the acute phase has ended, usually with hospital discharge, that issues such as drug dependence should be addressed. The acute postoperative period is often a time during which patients increase their drug manipulation and drug-seeking behaviors. For this reason it is important that only one team be responsible for the management of acute postoperative pain, and that trust and cooperation exist between all the members of the surgical and medical teams.

■ Extrinsic factors

The extrinsic factors that affect patient response to a particular protocol of acute pain management may also depend upon the type of surgery and the appropriateness of anesthesia and/or analgesia during surgery.

The type of surgery is often an important predictor of the intensity and duration of postoperative pain. It is well established that surgery involving soft tissues produces pain of a lower intensity than surgery involving bone resections. However, within the same orthopedic procedure the expected duration and intensity of the acute postoperative pain varies greatly among patients. For example, the duration of acute postoperative pain in a patient who undergoes total hip, ankle, or elbow replacement does not generally exceed 24–36 hours and the intensity is in most cases mild to moderate. In contrast, the acute postoperative pain associated with either total knee or shoulder replacement lasts for 48–72 hours and is frequently severe.

The extent of bone resections and rearrangements explains why many 'limited' foot surgeries are extremely painful, with pain lasting for more than 48 hours.

In this regard, patients with multiple trauma present particular challenges, not only because of the multiplicity of surgical sites, but also because multiple trauma generally reduces pain threshold in these patients. Accordingly, if the acute pain management protocols take into consideration the overall pain, the likelihood of the treatment being successful is low.

The importance of these preoperative conditions on the threshold of pain requires that the strategy of postoperative pain treatment be developed prior to surgery. Furthermore, it is important that regional anesthesia techniques (central or peripheral nerve blocks) be performed preoperatively, as well as the administration of COX2 inhibitors. N-Methyl-D-aspartate (NMDA)

receptor inhibitors, such as ketamine, have also been shown to reduce the requirement for pain medication postoperatively and should also be considered.

The therapeutic approach to acute postoperative pain management should be multimodal and take into account the expected duration and intensity of the postoperative pain. In this regard, any upper and lower orthopedic surgery associated with postoperative pain that lasts for more than 24 hours justifies continuous perineural infusion of local anesthetics. Major surgery involving the knee, shoulder, and ankle, and also open reduction and internal fixation of the ankle, femur, tibia, and upper extremity fractures, clearly justify continuous peripheral nerve blocks. The indications for continuous perineural infusions for total hip replacement remain controversial. However, we do believe, based on the literature and our clinical experience, that continuous peripheral nerve blocks are also indicated for hip replacement.

Since local anesthetics have an intrinsic toxic potential, choosing the least toxic one is especially important, particularly when high rates and long duration of the perineural infusion are likely. Lidocaine (lignocaine) has been used based on these principles. However, in orthopedic patients a selective sensory block is preferred to optimize early active physical therapy and so improve functional outcome. Since lidocaine produces both sensory and motor blocks, it does not seem the best choice. For several years bupivacaine has been the local anesthetic of choice. However, in the past few years ropivacaine has gained recognition. Borgeat et al. (2001) recently demonstrated that ropivacaine 0.2% provided a more selective sensory block than bupivacaine 0.15%, both via interscalene infusions, in patients who underwent open shoulder surgery.

Although the use of continuous perineural infusion forms the basis of our strategy for acute postoperative orthopedic pain management, our multimodal approach also includes cold therapy, COX2 inhibitors (started before surgery) and oral opioids such as oxycodone and sustained-release oxycodone. Our protocol includes the administration of 50 mg rofecoxib before surgery followed by 50 mg every day of rofecoxib starting on the day of surgery and continuing until discharge. COX2 inhibitors are now administered orally; however, new intravenous formulations of these drugs are being developed, which could be very interesting in the future. In most cases, we add a patient-controlled analgesia (PCA) morphine (1 mg/10 minutes, total dose of 6 mg/h without basal infusion) for the first night. If the patient requires more than 10 mg of morphine during the first postoperative day, on the second day we add 20 mg of sustained-release oxycodone q12h, along with oxycodone 5 mg q4h *pro re nata*. If morphine consumption during the first postoperative day is minimal, we add oxycodone 5 mg q4h *pro re nata* for break-through pain.

Finally, we recommend giving a bolus (8–10 ml) of local anesthetic solution through the catheter 20–30 minutes before physical therapy or to give the patients some oxycodone to allow pain-free exercising.

■ Techniques for continuous nerve blocks

The repeated injection technique was the first method used to prolong peripheral nerve blocks. Ansbro (1946) initially described a continuous brachial block technique based on the initial injection of 40 ml of procaine 1% followed by repeated injections to a total of 120–220 ml for 1.5–4 hours. Similarly, Manriquez and Pallares (1978) injected 20 ml of bupivacaine 0.25–0.5% every 6 hours via an interscalene catheter. Brands and Callanan (1978) preferred the injection of a 15–20 ml bolus of bupivacaine 0.5% with epinephrine (adrenaline) on demand via a lumbar plexus catheter after an initial injection of a 30 ml dose. Rosenblatt (1980) injected 15 ml of bupivacaine 0.75% via a femoral catheter every 6 hours for the first postoperative day and bupivacaine 0.5% at 4 ml/h for the second postoperative day. More recently, Chudinov et al. (1999) injected 2 mg/kg of bupivacaine 0.25% with epinephrine via a lumbar plexus catheter followed by additional injections (1–2 mg/kg) of the same mixture every 8 hours.

This repeated injection technique, based on the injection of a variable volume of local anesthetic mixture at various time intervals, remained prevalent until the introduction of continuous infusion pumps in the 1970s.

After the introduction of continuous infusion pumps, continuous perineural infusion of local anesthetic solution became prevalent for postoperative analgesia in patients with perineural catheters. Rosenblatt et al. (1979) used a continuous axillary infusion of bupivacaine

0.25% at 10 ml/h for 2 days. Smith et al. (1984) infused, via a sciatic catheter, a solution of bupivacaine 0.5% at 3 ml/h for 48 hours after an initial bolus of 10 ml of bupivacaine 0.75%. Dahl et al. (1988) infused bupivacaine 0.25% (0.35 mg/kg/h for 16 hours) via a lumbar plexus catheter after an initial bolus of 2 mg/kg of bupivacaine 0.5%. Anker-Moller et al. (1990) infused bupivacaine 0.125 or 0.25% at 0.14 mg/kg/h for 16 hours after a bolus of 0.4 mg/kg of bupivacaine 0.25 or 0.5%, respectively, via a lumbar plexus catheter. In this study, patients also received 1.5 g of acetylsalicylic acid rectally q6h. Mansour and Bennetts (1996) used a femoral continuous infusion of bupivacaine 0.125% with fentanyl 2 µg/ml at a rate of 10 ml/h for 28 hours. Morris and Lang (1997) first injected a bolus of bupivacaine 0.375% followed by an infusion of bupivacaine 0.1% at 8 ml/h for 48 hours via a parasacral catheter. In 1997, Singelyn et al. reported on the use of bupivacaine 0.125% plus 0.1 µg/ml sufentanil and 1 µg/ml clonidine infused via a popliteal catheter at a rate of 7 ml/h for 48 hours. Patients also received 1 g proparacetamol i.v. followed by 10–20 mg piritramide intramuscularly (i.m.). Singelyn et al. (1998) infused via a femoral catheter the same mixture at a rate of 10 ml/h for 48 hours. In this study, patients also received 1 g proparacetamol i.v. followed by 10–20 mg piritramide i.m. to optimize the postoperative pain treatment. Ganapathy et al. (1999) infused a solution of bupivacaine 0.1 and 0.2% at a rate of 10 ml/h for 48 hours via a fascia iliac catheter after an initial bolus of 30 ml of the same solution. Capdevilla et al. (1999) infused lidocaine 1%

with 2 μg/ml clonidine and 0.03 mg/ml morphine via a femoral catheter at a rate of 0.1 ml/kg/min after an initial bolus of 25 ml of lidocaine 2% as well as 0.1 mg/kg of morphine subcutaneously q6h *pro re nata*.

More recently, the introduction of PCA techniques for morphine and epidural analgesia led to the same concept being applied to continuous peripheral nerve block techniques.

In 1999 and 2001 Singelyn et al. compared the different approaches to continuous femoral nerve block, including a continuous infusion at 10 ml/h, a basal infusion of 5 ml/h with a bolus of 2.5 ml and a lockout period of 30 minutes (total 10 ml/h), and finally a patient-controlled infusion with no basal infusion and only 5 ml boluses with a lockout period of 30 minutes (total 10 ml/h). They concluded that a basal rate of 5 ml/h combined with a bolus of 2.5 ml and a lockout period of 30 minutes was the most appropriate technique, resulting in the lowest consumption of local anesthetic solution. Borgeat et al. (2000) reported similar results when evaluating a continuous interscalene brachial plexus block for shoulder surgery, and suggested the use of a continuous infusion rate of 5 ml/h with 3–4 ml boluses every 20 minutes.

In summary, three different approaches to continuous peripheral nerve block can be used:

- boluses of local anesthetic solution injected at fixed times by the team managing the patient's pain.
- continuous perineural infusion at a predetermined infusion rate, with no possibility of further implementation; and
- patient-controlled perineural anal-

gesia with a basal infusion rate of 2–5 ml/h and a bolus of 2–5 ml with a lockout period between 15 and 30 minutes for a total of 10–18 ml/h.

■ Indications

In recent years peripheral nerve blocks enjoyed a considerable resurgence of interest in both Europe and the USA, especially in the area of perineural continuous infusion (Todd and Brown 1999, Enneking and Wedel 2000). This was brought about by the availability of new local anesthetics, such as ropivacaine, and of electronic patient-controlled pumps.

Although single blocks are very effective for postoperative pain control in orthopedic patients, their effectiveness is limited by their duration, which does not exceed 14–18 hours. Intra-articular injections of local anesthetics or opioids have also been considered, but they have the same limitations as single blocks. Most inpatient and ambulatory orthopedic procedures for upper and lower extremities require more than 24 hours postoperative pain control. Consequently, single blocks and intra-articular injections do not cover the acute postoperative period effectively.

The recent increase in the use of low molecular weight heparin (LMWH) to prevent deep venous thrombosis and pulmonary emboli in orthopedic patients during the postoperative period (Stulberg et al. 1984, Leclerc et al. 1996, Heit et al. 1997) has considerably limited the use of a neuroaxial block for postoperative analgesia in orthopedic patients. In the USA, many institutions have banned the use of epidural analgesia in patients who

are scheduled to receive LMWH postoperatively, because of the fear of epidural hematoma, a rare complication (Horlocker and Wedel 1998a, Lumpkin 1998). Despite the development of guidelines (Heit et al. 1997, Horlocker and Wedel 1998b), there is no effective way to prevent the occurrence of postoperative epidural hematoma, a complication that carries with it a very serious risk of permanent nerve damage, including paraplegia. This situation has also contributed greatly to the increased interest in continuous perineural infusion techniques.

■ Continuous nerve blocks for total arthroplasty

Shoulder arthroplasty

Our protocol includes the preoperative placement of an interscalene catheter through a 37.5 mm insulated Tuohy needle connected to a nerve stimulator. Prior to surgery the patient also receives 50 mg of rofecoxib.

The surgery is conducted under sedation and/or light general anesthesia. After surgery the patients are connected to an infusion of ropivacaine 0.2% at 8 ml/h for 48–72 hours, and PCA morphine (1 mg with a lockout period of 10 minutes for a total of 6 mg with no basal). Immediately after surgery the patients also receive another 50 mg of rofecoxib. The next morning, the patients are evaluated for the intensity of the motor and sensory blocks as well as for the amount of morphine consumption. In most cases consumption is less than 10 mg, and a prescription of 5 mg oxycodone q4h *pro re nata* is added, along with discontinuation of PCA. If the consumption of morphine during the first 12 hours following surgery is greater than 10 mg, sustained-release oxycodone 20 mg q12h is added to the regimen (with PCA discontinued).

Knee arthroplasty

Femoral block. Several studies have demonstrated that the use of postoperative continuous femoral infusion is associated with a postoperative decrease in morphine consumption by up to 70% and associated side effects in patients who undergo total knee replacement (Mansour and Bennetts 1996, Singelyn et al. 1997, Capdevilla et al. 1999, Ganapathy et al. 1999, Chelly et al. 2001d). Hirst et al. (1996) reported a single femoral block with bupivacaine 0.5% to be as effective as a single block with bupivacaine 0.5% followed by continuous femoral infusion for total knee replacement. However, it is important to recognize that these authors used an infusion of bupivacaine 0.125% at 6 ml/h, which other studies have demonstrated to be below the therapeutic threshold (Ganapathy et al. 1999).

The continuous infusion of local anesthetics is associated with a faster postoperative functional recovery (Singelyn et al. 1998), better immediate and secondary functional outcomes, and a substantial reduction of length of hospital stay (Chelly 2001d) and time for rehabilitation (Capdevilla et al. 1999). Our data also indicate that continuous femoral infusions are associated with blood-sparing effects and a related decrease in the number of postoperative blood transfusions compared with PCA morphine and

epidural analgesia (Chelly et al. 2001d).

Our current protocol includes a preoperative posterior sciatic block to also block the posterior femoral nerve of the thigh and prevent tourniquet pain. A femoral block, using a 50 mm insulated Tuohy needle and a nerve stimulator, is then performed, followed by the placement of 20-gauge femoral catheter 10–12 cm at the skin. The femoral block is completed, if required, by blocking the obturator and the lateral femoral cutaneous nerves. Prior to surgery the patient also receives 50 mg of rofecoxib. The surgery is conducted under sedation. Recently, we have preferred dexmedetomidine, because it produces sedation without respiratory depression, and it is also analgesic. After surgery, the patient is connected to an infusion of ropivacaine 0.2% at 10 ml/h, a PCA morphine (1 mg with a lockout period of 10 minutes for a total of 6 mg with no basal). The patients also receive 50 mg of rofecoxib after surgery and every day until discharge. The next morning, the patient is evaluated for pain, intensity of motor and sensory blocks, and recovery of the sciatic block, while the amount of morphine consumption is recorded. In most cases the consumption is less than 10 mg, so a prescription of 5 mg oxycodone q4h *pro re nata* is added and PCA morphine is discontinued. If the consumption of morphine during the first 24 hours following surgery is greater than 10 mg, then 20 mg sustained-release oxycodone q12h is added to the regimen. In these patients most of the postoperative pain is located behind the knee and is of sciatic distribution.

Lumbar plexus block. Although the use of a continuous lumbar plexus infusion represents an interesting alternative for the postoperative management of pain in patients who undergo total knee replacement, it seems that the posterior approach is not performed as often as the anterior approach.

Hip arthroplasty

Although Singelyn et al. (2001) recently reported the use of continuous femoral infusions for postoperative pain control after hip replacement, continuous lumbar plexus block seems more appropriate. Furthermore, the postoperative pain associated with total hip replacement is of a mild-to-severe intensity in most patients only during the first 24–36 hours; for this reason single blocks have also been recommended (Stevens et al. 2000). However, we believe that continuous infusion techniques are indicated for the control of mild-to-severe pain lasting more than 24 hours in orthopedic patients. Therefore, our patients who undergo total hip replacement also benefit from continuous perineural infusions of local anesthetic for 36 hours. Although we prefer to use a lumbar plexus approach in this setting, our experience with continuous femoral infusions has also been satisfactory.

Our protocol includes the placement of a lumbar plexus block using a 100 mm insulated Tuohy needle followed by the placement of a catheter. A posterior sciatic block is also performed preoperatively to minimize the impact of the possible postoperative sciatic pain. The patient also receives 50 mg of rofecoxib prior to surgery and then every day after surgery until discharge. The next morning, the patient is evaluated for the intensity of motor and sensory blocks and for the recovery of the sciatic block, and the amount of morphine consumption is recorded. If morphine consumption during the first day after surgery is less than 10 mg, 5 mg oral oxycodone q4h *pro re nata* is added and PCA morphine is discontinued; otherwise sustained-release oxycodone 20 mg q12h is added to the regimen (with PCA discontinued).

Ankle arthroplasty

Our current protocol includes a preoperative femoral or sapheneous block along with a lateral sciatic block placed with a 100 mm insulated Tuohy needle and a nerve stimulator, followed by the placement of a catheter. Prior to surgery the patient also receives 50 mg of rofecoxib. The surgery is conducted under sedation or light general anesthesia. After surgery the patient is connected to an infusion of ropivacaine 0.2% at 10 ml/h, and to PCA morphine. The patient also receives another 50 mg of rofecoxib after surgery and every day until discharge. The next morning, the patient is evaluated for pain, intensity of the motor and sensory blocks, and recovery of the sciatic block, and the amount of morphine consumed is recorded. Discontinuation of PCA morphine is based on morphine consumption during the first day after surgery, and it is replaced with 5 mg oral oxycodone q4h *pro re nata* or sustained-release oxycodone 20 mg q12h. Most patients are discharged on the second postoperative day and go home with ambulatory pumps that allow

them to continue the postoperative sciatic continuous infusion of ropivacaine for another 48 hours.

Elbow reconstruction

This surgery is associated with a mild postoperative pain that does not exceed 24–36 hours. Therefore, the use of a single axillary block may be indicated. We prefer a continuous technique along with the placement of a catheter, using Raj's infraclavicular approach (Raj et al. 1973). As previously discussed for continuous infusion, the patients receive 50 mg rofecoxib prior to and after surgery and every day for 8–10 days. Patients are usually discharged on the second or third day.

■ Continuous nerve blocks for trauma patients

The use of continuous peripheral blocks is especially interesting in trauma patients, in whom pain is often combined with a decrease of local blood flow. In this regard, the continuous infusion of local anesthetics adds analgesia to the concomitant block of sympathetic fibers, which produces local vasodilation and favors peripheral circulation.

For upper extremity trauma, the indication for perineural continuous infusion techniques is based not only on the intensity and expected duration of the postoperative pain, but also on the potential benefit associated with local vasodilation, especially cases of reimplantation.

Irrespective of the specific indications, our protocol includes a multimodal approach based on the use of COX2 inhibitors (rofecoxib 50 mg every day), and continuous infusion of ropivacaine 0.2% at a rate that

varies from 6 to 10 ml/h. These protocols are complemented with long-lasting opioids, such as sustained-release oxycodone (20 mg q12h), and muscle relaxants, such as cyclobenzaprine (Flexeril) 10 mg q8h, because of the associated muscle spasm with trauma. Since many trauma patients are often depressed, the early prescription of a tricyclic antidepressor is also beneficial, as is the use of gabapentin (Neurontin) in cases of traumatic amputation. Finally, it is very important to ensure that these patients can sleep at night, and the appropriate medication needs to be prescribed.

Upper limb

The type of injury, its location, and the nerves involved usually determine the catheter location, as well as the associated medical conditions. Thus, an interscalene catheter may be placed for injury of the forearm and the hand (except if an ulnar nerve block is also required), especially when the injury involves the median with or without the radial nerve. In contrast, a hand injury that involves the ulnar nerve rarely benefits from a continuous interscalene technique. Injury that involves the humerus and elbow may also benefit from either an interscalene or an axillary continuous block. The ability to move the injured limb may also dictate the approach used for the continuous technique. Indeed, for a patient not able to abduct the arm, a supra- and/or infraclavicular technique may be preferred. The expected duration of continuous infusion may also contribute to the choice of technique: for a prolonged continuous axillary block (more than 3 days) it is preferable to place an axillary catheter using the Raj infracla-vicular approach rather than the classic axillary approach. Interscalene catheters are also difficult to maintain in place beyond 3–4 days, even though tunneling them helps.

Lower limb

Acetabular fracture. An acetabular fracture is the only condition in which we perform a block in an anesthetized patient at the end of surgery, while the patient is still in a lateral position. Our protocol includes the location of the lumbar plexus using a 100 mm insulated Tuohy needle and a nerve stimulator. After the needle is positioned correctly, 30 ml of ropivacaine 0.75% or 0.5% or a mixture of mepivacaine 1.5% and ropivacaine 0.75% (v/v) are injected, followed by the placement of a 20-gauge catheter 10–12 cm at the skin. Following surgery the catheter is infused with ropivacaine 0.2% at 10 ml/h for 48 hours, with PCA morphine. The patient is also given 50 mg of rofecoxib preoperatively and every day until discharge. The day after surgery PCA morphine is discontinued and replaced with sustained-release oxycodone (20 mg q12h) along with oxycodone (5 mg q4h *pro re nata*). With this technique patients are able to ambulate within the first 36–48 hours after surgery.

Hip fracture. Continuous lumbar plexus block has been reported as an effective technique to control pre- and postoperative pain in patients with a femoral neck fracture (Brands and Callanan 1978, Chudinov et al. 1999). Different protocols based on the use of a psoas compartment approach

have been suggested. Brands and Callanan used an initial injection of 30 ml of bupivacaine 0.5% with epinephrine followed by 15 ml of the same mixture every 4–6 hours. Chudinov et al. recommended an initial injection of 2 mg/kg of bupivacaine 0.25% with epinephrine followed by additional injections of 1–2 mg/kg of the same mixture every 8 hours.

Our protocol includes the placement of a lumbar plexus block with 30 ml of ropivacaine 0.5–0.75% or mepivacaine 1.5% and ropivacaine 0.75% (v/v) followed by the placement of a 20-gauge catheter 10–12 cm at the skin. Following surgery the catheter is infused with ropivacaine 0.2% at 10 ml/h for 36 hours, with PCA morphine. The patient also receives a COX2 inhibitor until discharge, while the day after surgery PCA morphine is usually substituted by sustained-release oxycodone (20 mg q12h) associated with oxycodone (5 mg q4h *pro re nata*). With this technique patients are able to ambulate within the first 18–24 hours after surgery.

Femur fracture. Open reduction and internal fixation of a femur fracture can benefit greatly from either a continuous femoral or a posterior lumbar plexus block. The choice of the technique depends on the mobility of the patient, importance of the femoral hematoma, location of the fracture, and relationship between the femoral nerve and the site of the fracture. Prior to surgery, often a catheter is placed in the femoral sheath using an anterior approach. Either a femoral or a lumbar plexus approach can be used when the catheter is placed after surgery. The expected pain in these patients is mostly mild and lasts less

than 48 hours. Furthermore, rarely is immediate postoperative physical therapy required. Therefore, the use of continuous ropivacaine 0.3% at 8–10 ml/h for 48 hours may be indicated.

Patella fracture. Open reduction and internal fixation of a patella fracture is exquisitely painful at rest after surgery. Furthermore, these patients need to be mobilized immediately after surgery to maximize the functional outcome, and thus good control of pain on exercise is a crucial goal. Although a lumbar plexus infusion might be indicated, we prefer a continuous femoral infusion with ropivacaine 0.2% at 8–10 ml/h. Usually these patients benefit from the use of continuous passive motion (CPM) machines within the first few hours after surgery. They are often discharged the next day with an ambulatory pump to maintain a sensory femoral block for another couple of days.

Fracture of tibial plateau. Open reduction and internal fixation of a tibial plateau fracture is moderately to mildly painful postoperatively at rest. However, these patients need to be mobilized immediately after surgery to maximize the functional outcome. For this reason proper control of pain on exercise (CPM) is crucial. A subgluteal or lateral sciatic approach is indicated and a continuous sciatic infusion with ropivacaine 0.2% at 6–8 ml/h for 48 hours is often enough. However, since the medial aspect of the leg is not blocked, which depends on the sapheneous nerve, it is necessary to inform the patient and implement the analgesic regimen with an appropriate oral medication (COX2 inhibitor and opioids). As for any continuous sciatic block, it is important to recognize that these patients must be monitored closely for physical symptoms of the compartment syndrome, which usually occurs in the sciatic territory. These patients are generally not candidates for an ambulatory continuous infusion technique.

Tibial fracture. A tibial fracture rarely requires a continuous sciatic block for more than 36 hours. Again, in these patients a subgluteal or lateral sciatic approach is indicated. Furthermore, these patients are mobilized early and therefore benefit from the use of ropivacaine 0.2%. As mentioned above, they may complain of pain in the medial aspect of the leg if an appropriate multimodal approach is not used.

Ankle and calcaneous fractures. Open reduction and internal fixation of an ankle and, even more so, of a calcaneum fracture are often associated with severe and prolonged postoperative pain. However, the requirement for active postoperative physical therapy is usually limited, which allows the use of ropivacaine 0.3% at 6–8 ml/h, along with rofecoxib 50 mg every day and sustained-release oxycodone 20 mg q12h.

Continuous nerve blocks for amputation

Peripheral nerve blocks and postoperative continuous perineural infusions represent interesting techniques for patients who undergo amputations. Although a number of patients require upper and lower limb amputation for tumors, in most cases peripheral vascular dis-

ease is the main indication for amputation of the lower extremity. Consequently, most of these patients are elderly and have multiple organ failures, including renal, cardiac, and respiratory failure. They also are quite often on anticoagulants.

A combined sciatic and lumbar plexus block, or preferably a femoral block if the patient is on anticoagulants, satisfies the requirement for surgery. Furthermore, for amputation above the knee a femoral catheter is placed preoperatively for postoperative infusion. In contrast, for amputation below the knee a lateral sciatic or subgluteus catheter is indicated. Postoperative pain control includes a continuous perineural infusion of ropivacaine 0.3% at 6–8 ml/h for 5 days. Often a muscle relaxant [cyclobenzaprine (Flexeril) 10 mg q8h] is also prescribed, along with PCA morphine until the morning after surgery. As previously discussed, sustained-release oxycodone 20 mg q12h along with 5 mg oxycodone for break-through pain usually substitutes PCA morphine on the day after surgery. Particular attention is given to the development of phantom pain syndrome. The occurrence of such a complication, which is rare in our practice during the immediate postoperative period, responds very well to gabapentin (Neurontin) 300 mg q8h as a starting dose. In the absence of hypovolemia, the patient also receives 50 mg of rofecoxib prior to and after the surgery and then every day.

For upper extremity amputation, the approach chosen depends on the level at which the amputation is performed. The placement of an interscalene or supraclavicular

catheter is indicated for amputation at the level of the shoulder. Below the shoulder, an axillary or infraclavicular approach may be better.

Continuous nerve blocks and intra-articular infusions for outpatients

There is a constant search for techniques that enable increased postoperative pain control, especially after ambulatory orthopedic surgery. In addition, the introduction of health maintenance organizations, managed care organizations, and particular methods for reimbursement by organizations such as Medicare Diagnosis Related Group (DRG) led to a reduction in the period of hospitalization. In this regard, Pavlin et al. (1998) showed that a peripheral nerve block as the sole anesthesia technique reduces the length of hospital stay for outpatient procedures by more than 1 hour, but single injection blocks produce postoperative pain control for a short period only.

To extend the postoperative analgesic properties of peripheral nerve blocks, continuous perineural blocks have also been considered for outpatient surgery. Furthermore, over the past few years small disposable and non-disposable pumps for continuous infusions have been introduced. There are two different types:

• The first type is disposable and elastomeric (I-Flow, Lake Forest, CA, USA; Baxter, New Providence, NJ, USA). These pumps deliver either one rate of infusion (2, 5, or 10 ml/h) or a bolus of 2 ml over a 20 minute period. They have various capacities according to the rate of infusion

(50 ml for 2 ml/h, 100 ml for 5 ml/h, and 250 ml for 10 ml/h).

- The second type is an electronic pump (Sorenson Medical, West Jordan, UT, USA). It allows a choice of the basal rate of infusion (0–30 ml/h), the volume of a bolus (0–20 ml), and the lockout period (0–24 hours). In addition, these pumps have an alarm system that detects dysfunctions of the pump and corrects them.

It is important, especially for ambulatory cases, to recognize that local anesthetics have an intrinsic toxic potential and, therefore, should be used at the minimum required dose to minimize the risk of systemic toxicity. Furthermore, the bags that contain local anesthetic mixtures have a maximum capacity of 250 ml and there is a direct relationship between the rate of infusion and the possible duration of infusion that a given volume can provide. Therefore, the smaller the volume that is basally infused the longer the pump can run. Singelyn et al. (1999) and Borgeat et al. (2000) demonstrated that PCA pumps provide the same postoperative pain control as continuous infusion with a lower volume for inpatients. Grant et al. (2001) used continuous sciatic infusions at 10 ml/h with a 250 ml elastomeric pump that ran for only 25 hours. In contrast, Chelly et al. (2001a, 2001b) used a basal infusion rate of 5 ml/h combined with a patient-controlled bolus of 2 ml and a lockout time of 15 minutes, which provided postoperative pain control for almost 48 hours. Irrespective of the type of pump (elastomeric or electronic) and the mode of administration (continuous, or PCA with or without basal infusion), if the duration of infusion requires a larger volume the capacity of the bag can be increased up to 500 ml by either using a larger bag or by connecting two bags.

We are using perineural infusions of local anesthetics in ambulatory patients with femoral, subgluteal, lateral sciatic, axillary, and interscalene catheters who have had patella repair, anterior cruciate ligament (ACL) repair, foot surgery, and upper extremity surgery, including hand, elbow, and shoulder surgery. When using this technique it is important to select the patient appropriately. Although some of the criteria listed below are still under discussion, such as the distance between the hospital and the patient's home, others are accepted by most of the users including:

- acceptance of the technique by the patient;
- ability of the patient and significant others to be educated and understand how to use the pump, to recognize the early symptoms of local anesthetic toxicity (sedation, nausea, vomiting, metallic taste, etc.), and to look for bleeding, inflammation, or infection at the insertion site during the infusion and after the catheter has been removed;
- assurance that someone will be with the patient during the postoperative period; and
- ability to reach a member of the acute orthopedic pain service in case of a problem or questions that arise (to have at least one telephone in the house).

The patient must also be instructed what to do when the catheter needs to be removed. In France, where anesthesiologists are starting to use this technique, a home-care nurse visits the patient at home twice a day.

In our practice, patients are called at least twice a day to verify the efficacy of pain relief and that there are no associated side effects. We have rarely been called by the patient, but when we were it was always about pump dysfunction. The rate of infusion, bolus, and lockout period are set prior to the patient's discharge. All patients are discharged with a diary and a request that the patient record the degree of pain with a visual analog score (VAS) every 4 hours, except during the night. Patients are also given an appropriate telephone and pager number to allow them to reach a member of the acute orthopedic pain team 24 hours a day. In every case, the continuous perineural block for ambulatory orthopedic surgery is part of a multimodal approach. All of our patients are also discharged with a prescription for 10 days of a COX2 inhibitor (rofecoxib 50 mg, except in the presence of contraindications) and opioids. The potency of the opioids varies according to the expected postoperative pain (sustained-released oxicodone/oxycodone for patella repair versus hydrocodone for ACL) to minimize postoperative pain and maximize early functional recovery.

Mallon and Thomas (2000) demonstrated the benefit of PCA wound infusion in patients undergoing shoulder surgery. Savoie et al. (2000) demonstrated that continuous subacromial infusions of local anesthetics for 48 hours at 2 ml/h using an elastomeric spring-loaded pump provided some postoperative analgesia. We recently studied, in the same group of patients, the effects of 3 ml/h with boluses of 2 ml every 15 ml using a PCA pump and found similar results to those previously published. However, the preliminary data suggest that postoperative subacromial and/or intra-articular infusions of ropivacaine 0.2% at a basal rate of 5 ml/h with boluses of 2 ml and a lockout period of 15 minutes using a PCA pump may provide better postoperative analgesia.

■ Conclusions

Continuous peripheral nerve blocks are indicated for both inpatient and outpatient orthopedic procedures and allow safe and fast recovery. However, these techniques need to account appropriately for the postoperative require-

ment of active physical therapy. The duration of infusion varies with the type of surgery and the expected duration of postoperative pain. Finally, the optimum use of these techniques is as part of a multimodal approach to postoperative pain management.

CHAPTER 3

COMPLICATIONS

J.E. Chelly

Complications of continuous peripheral nerve blocks

In his original article, Ansbro (1946) reported three cases of sweating and pallor in the 27 patients who benefited from a continuous supraclavicular technique, although the author did not attribute these symptoms to local anesthetic toxicity. However, very few cases of local anesthetic toxicity have been reported with continuous anesthetic techniques. This is most likely because with the continuous infusion technique low concentrations of local anesthetic solution are usually used and the rate of infusion rarely exceeds 10 ml/h.

To assess the complications associated with continuous infusion techniques, we reviewed 58 different published articles that described more than 2000 patients who had benefited from continuous perineural infusions. This review demonstrated that the overall frequency of complications was extremely low. Although most of the authors intended to report any associated complication, the majority of them did not observe any severe complication. Among the 58 articles reviewed only 15 reported complications. Brands and Callanan (1978), who studied the use of a continuous psoas compartment block in patients with hip fractures,

reported one death, which at autopsy was related to an acute myocardial infarction. It is well established that postoperative myocardial infarction is not an unusual complication in elderly patients who undergo major orthopedic surgery. Other reported complications are similar to those for single injection techniques, such as a few cases of a decrease (within 10% of baseline values) in blood pressure, hoarseness and Bernard–Horner syndrome, phrenic paresis, and major hypoxia that requires oxygen therapy after interscalene catheter placement. Excessive motor weakness has been reported following interscalene catheter placement, while tenderness at the site has been reported with a frequency of 15% for psoas compartment blocks. Singelyn et al. (1999) demonstrated that the frequency of these side effects was reduced with patient-controlled perineural administration of local anesthetic compared to a continuous infusion mode for a similar overall volume per hour.

Matsuda et al. (1982) reported one pneumothorax after a supraclavicular catheter in 49 patients, and one paresthesia of the forearm that resolved after 1 month. Sada et al. (1983), in the largest published series with 597 axillary catheters, reported three cases of nerve injury (0.25%), seven cases of systemic toxic reaction (2.85%), and one

important hematoma that limited perfusion. In 1996, Ribeiro et al. reported two cases of brachial plexus reversible irritation by an interscalene catheter. Cook (1991) reported one case of epidural catheterization after the placement of an interscalene catheter.

Selander (1977) reported 33 cases with puncture of a blood vessel out of 137 axillary catheters studied. However, this complication did not affect patient outcome, except for one compressive hematoma.

With respect to nerve injuries, it is important to recognize that:

- the frequency of nerve injuries reported with continuous perineural techniques is very small (less than 3/2000 patients); and
- nerve damage related to patient positioning and the surgery itself, especially for orthopedic surgery, is far more frequent than nerve injuries associated with peripheral nerve blocks.

When a patient who has received a single injection block and/or continuous infusion develops motor deficit in the territory of the block after surgery, an early nerve conduction study usually enables differentiation between surgical and anesthetic causes.

More specific to the placement of a catheter is the incidence of catheter kinking, which required the placement of another catheter in eight patients (Selander 1977), as well as displacement of the catheter in six of 60 interscalene catheters (Haasio et al. 1990, Borgeat et al. 1997). Singelyn and Gouverneur (1999) reported their experience with 1142 femoral catheters; they recorded a total of 5.5% catheter-related problems (1.6% kinked and 3.9% displaced). Johnson (1994) reported that continuous femoral infusion in children was associated with leaking, but did not prevent continuation of the perineural infusion. The same author also reported one case of localized infection after 4 days of infusion. Although in most cases the catheters were maintained for 2–3 days, cases of catheters maintained for more than 10 days have been published with no associated systemic infection. Chudinov et al. (1999) also reported three patients with local erythema.

Our experience, based on more than a thousand perineural and/or intra-articular catheters (including interscalene, axillary, infraclavicular, lumbar plexus, femoral, and sciatic catheters), is consistent with the literature. We have not observed any nerve deficit related to this technique, nor have we experienced any systemic or local infection. Our catheters are monitored at least once a day every day, and they are maintained in place

from 36 hours (femoral or lumbar plexus for total hip replacement) up to 5–6 days (especially after amputation).

Although the use of tunneled catheters decreases the frequency of catheter displacement, interscalene, axillary, and even lumbar plexus catheters may be difficult to maintain in place for more than 48 or 72 hours. Leaking of the catheter at the insertion site is the most frequent complication (<10%), but it is rarely a reason for discontinuing the infusion. Less frequent is disconnection of the tip of the catheter, but this is also of minor consequence, since the catheter connector can be easily replaced.

The integrity of the catheter must be verified every day, and in all cases when the catheter is removed. In our experience we have observed only one case of a catheter with a knot at the time of removal. This was a femoral catheter that was introduced 15 cm beyond the tip of the needle. After this case, we decided to limit the length to which the catheter is introduced to 3–4 cm. The Seldinger technique or a metallic guided catheter may allow the catheter to be introduced further. However, the benefit of these technical variations remains to be demonstrated.

Although not directly related to placement of the catheter, when reviewing complications those associated with the use of a pump should be considered.

These include pump failure, disconnection of the pump and the catheter, and (the most frequent problem) keeping a filled bag at all times. When a patient with a continuous catheter complains of pain in the associated region, the most frequent reason is not a failed block but an empty local anesthetic bag not replaced on time. We cannot stress enough that the effectiveness of these techniques depends upon the coordination of different health care givers, including the attendant nurse, the pharmacist, and the physical therapist. If appropriate provision is not made to account for an increase in pain prior to the beginning of physical therapy, the patient will experience pain unnecessarily. Providing a bolus (5–10 ml) of local anesthetic solution 20–30 minutes before starting the physical therapy can easily prevent this. Similarly, if appropriate provision is not made to order the next local anesthetic bag, the patient can remain without infusions for hours. Finally, new batteries must be immediately available, especially when infusions run for several days.

References

Ang ET, Lassale B, Goldfarb G.
*Continuous axillary brachial plexus
block – a clinical and anatomical study.
Anesth Analg, 1984; 63: 680–684.*

Anker-Moller E, Spansberg N, Dahl JB,
Christensen E, Schultz P, Carlsson P.
*Continuous blockade of the lumbar plexus
after knee surgery: a comparison of the
plasma concentrations and analgesic effect
of bupivacaine 0.250% and 0.125%.
Acta Anaesthesiol Scand, 1990; 34:
468–472.*

Ansbro FP.
*A method of continuous brachial plexus block.
Am J Surg, 1946; 71: 716–722.*

Ben-David, B, Lee E, Croitoru M.
*Psoas block for surgical repair of hip fracture:
a case report and description of a catheter
technique.
Anesth Analg, 1990; 71: 298–301.*

Borgeat A, Schappi B, Biasca N, Gerber C.
*Patient-controlled analgesia after major
shoulder surgery.
Anesthesiology, 1997; 87: 1343–1347.*

Borgeat A, Perschak H, Bird P, Hodler J,
Gerber C.
*Patient-controlled interscalene analgesia
with ropivacaine 0.2% versus patient-
controlled intravenous analgesia after
major shoulder surgery.
Anesthesiology, 2000; 92: 102–108.*

Borgeat A, Kalberer F, Jacob H, Ruetsch YA,
Gerber C.
*Patient-controlled interscalene analgesia
with ropivacaine 0.2% versus bupivacaine
0.15% after major open shoulder surgery:
the effects on hand motor function.
Anesth Analg, 2001; 92: 218–223.*

Brands E, Callanan VI.
*Continuous lumbar plexus block – analgesia
for femoral neck fractures.
Anaesth Intens Care, 1978; 6: 256–258.*

Capdevilla X, Barthelet Y, Biboulet P,
Ryckwaert Y, Rubenovitch J, d'Athis F.
*Effects of perioperative analgesic technique
on the surgical outcome and duration
of rehabilitation after minor knee surgery.
Anesthesiology, 1999; 91: 8–15.*

Chelly JE, Greger J, Al-Samsam T,
Casati A, McGarvey W, Clanton TO.
*Continuous lateral sciatic infusions for
postoperative pain control after ankle surgery.
J Foot Ankle. Submitted, 2001a.*

Chelly JE, Gebhard R, Coupe K, Greger J,
Khan A.
*Local anesthetic PCA via a femoral catheter
for the postoperative pain control of an ACL
performed as an outpatient procedure.
Am J Anesthesiology, 2001b; 28: 192–194.*

Chelly JE, Greger J, Casati A, et al.
*Continuous lumbar plexus block for acute
postoperative pain management after
open reduction and internal fixation
of acetabular fractures.
J Orthopaedic Trauma, 2001c; in press.*

Chelly JE, Greger J, Gebhard R, et al.
*Continuous femoral blocks improve
recovery and outcome of patients undergoing
total knee arthroplasty.
J Arthroplasty, 2001d; 16:436–445.*

Chudinov A, Berkenstadt H, Salai M,
Cahana A, Perel A.
*Continuous psoas compartment block
for anesthesia and perioperative analgesia
in patients with hip fractures.
Reg Anesth Pain Med, 1999; 4: 563–568.*

Cook LB.
*Unsuspected extradural catheterization in an
interscalene block.
Br J Anaesth, 1991; 67: 473–475.*

Dahl JB, Christiansen CL, Daugaard JJ,
Schultz P, Carlsson P.
*Continuous blockade of the lumbar plexus
after knee surgery – postoperative analgesia
and bupivacaine plasma concentrations.
A controlled clinical trial.
Anaesthesia, 1988; 43: 1015–1018.*

De Krey JA, Schroeder CF, Buechel DR.
*Continuous brachial plexus block.
Anesthesiology, 1969; 30: 332.*

Edwards ND, Wright EM,
*Continuous 3-in-1 nerve blockade
for postoperative pain relief after total
knee replacement.
Anesth Analg, 1992; 75: 265–267.*

Enneking RK, Wedel DJ.
*The art and science of peripheral nerve blocks.
Anesth Analg, 2000; 90: 1–2.*

Fewtrell MS, Sapsford DJ, Herrick MJ,
Noble-Jamieson G, Russell RI.
*Continuous axillary nerve block
for chronic pain.
Arch Dis Child, 1994; 70: 54–55.*

Ganapathy S, Wasserman RA, Watson JT,
et al.
*Modified continuous femoral three-in-one
block for postoperative pain after total
knee arthroplasty.
Anesth Analg, 1999; 89: 1197–1202.*

Grant SA, Nielsen KC, Greengrass RA,
Steele SM, Klein SM.
*Continuous peripheral nerve block
for ambulatory surgery.
Reg Anesth Pain Med, 2001; 26: 209–214.*

Haasio J, Tuominen M, Rosenberg PH.
*Continuous interscalene brachial plexus
block during and after shoulder surgery.
Ann Chir Gynaecol, 1990; 79: 103–107.*

Heit JA, Berkowitz SD, Bona R, et al.
*Efficacy and safety of low molecular weight
heparin (ardeparin sodium) compared
to warfarin for the prevention of venous
thromboembolism after total knee
replacement surgery: a double-blind,
dose-ranging study.
Thromb Haemost, 1997; 77: 32–38.*

Hirst GC, Lang SA, Dust WN, Cassidy JD,
Yip RW.
*Femoral nerve block. Single injection
versus continuous infusion for total knee
arthroplasty.
Reg Anesth, 1996; 21: 292–297.*

Horlocker TT, Wedel DJ.
*Anticoagulation and neuraxial block:
historical perspective, anesthetic implications,
and risk management.
Reg Anesth Pain Med, 1998a; 23: 129–134.*

Horlocker TT, Wedel DJ.
*Neuraxial block and low-molecular-weight
heparin: balancing perioperative analgesia
and thromboprophylaxis.
Reg Anesth Pain Med, 1998b; 23:
164–177.*

Iskandar H, Rakotondriamihary S,
Dixmerias F, Binje B, Maurette P.
*Analgésie par bloc axillaire continu après
chirurgie des traumatismes graves de la
main: auto-administration versus injection
continue.
Ann Fr Anesth Reanim, 1998; 17:
1099–1103.*

Johnson CM.
*Continuous femoral nerve blockade for
analgesia in children with femoral fractures.
Anaesth Intensive Care, 1994; 22:
281–283.*

Klein SM, D'Ercole F, Greengrass RA, Warner DS.
Enoxaprin associated with psoas hematoma and lumbar plexopathy after lumbar plexus block.
Anesthesiology, 1997; 87: 1576–1579.

Klein SM, Greengrass RA, Gleason DH, Nunley JA, Steele SM.
Major ambulatory surgery with continuous regional anesthesia and a disposable infusion pump.
Anesthesiology, 1999; 91: 563–565.

Leclerc JR, Geerts WH, Desjardins L, et al.
Prevention of venous thromboembolism after knee arthroplasty a randomized, double-blind trial comparing enoxaprin with warfarin.
Ann Intern Med, 1996; 124: 619–626.

Lumpkin MM.
FDA Public Health Advisory.
Letter to the Editor.
Anesthesiology, 1998; 88: 27–28A.

Mallon WJ, Thomas CW.
Patient-controlled lidocaine analgesia for acromioplasty surgery.
J Shoulder Elbow Surg, 2000; 9: 85–88.

Manriquez RG, Pallares V.
Continuous brachial plexus block for prolonged sympathectomy and control of pain.
Anesth Analg, 1978; 57: 128–130.

Mansour NY, Bennetts FE.
An observational study of combined continuous lumbar plexus and single-shot sciatic nerve blocks for post-knee surgery analgesia.
Reg Anesth, 1996; 21: 287–291.

Matsuda M, Kato N, Hosoi M.
Continuous brachial plexus block for replantation in the upper extremity.
Hand, 1982; 14: 129–134.

Morris GF, Lang SA.
Continuous parasacral sciatic nerve block: two case reports.
Reg Anesth, 1997; 22: 469–472.

Parkinson SK, Mueller JB, Little WB, Bailey SL.
Extent of blockade with various approaches to the lumbar plexus.
Anesth Analg, 1989; 68: 243–248.

Paut O, Sallabery M, Schreiber-Deturmeny E, Remond Ch, Bruguerolle B, Camboulives J.
Continuous fascia iliaca compartment block in children: A prospective evaluation of plasma bupivacaine concentrations, pain scores, and side effects.
Anesth Analg, 2001; 92: 1159–1163.

Pavlin DJ, Rapp SE, Polissar NL, Malµgren JA, Koerschgen M, Keyes H.
Factors affecting discharge time in adult outpatients.
Anesth Analg, 1998; 87: 816–826.

Pere P.
The effect of continuous interscalene brachial plexus block with 0.125% bupivacaine plus fentanyl on diaphragmatic motility and ventilatory function.
Reg Anesth, 1993; 18: 93–97.

Pere P, Pitkanen M, Rosenberg PH, et al.
Effect of continuous interscalene brachial plexus block on diaphragm motion and on ventilatory function.
Acta Anaesthesiol Scand, 1992; 36: 53–57.

Raj PP, Montgomery SJ, Nettle D, Jenkins MT.
Infraclavicular brachial plexus block – a new approach.
Anesth Analg 1973; 52: 897–903.

Rawal N.
Analgesia for day-case surgery.
Br J Anaesth, 2001; 87: 73–87.

Rawal N, Axelsson K, Hylander J.
Postoperative patient-controlled local anesthetic administration at home.
Anesth Analg, 1998; 86: 86–89.

Reuben SS, Connelly RR.
Postoperative analgesic effects of celecoxib or rofecoxib after spinal fusion surgery.
Anesth Analg, 2000; 91: 1221–1225.

Ribeiro FC, Georgousis H, Bertram R, Scheiberg G.
Plexus eritation caused by interscalene brachial plexus catheter for shoulder surgery.
Anesth Analg, 1996; 82: 870–872.

Rosenblatt R.
Continuous femoral anesthesia for lower extremity surgery.
Anesth Analg, 1980; 59: 631–632.

Rosenblatt R, Pepitone-Rockwell F, McKillop MJ.
Continuous axillary analgesia for traumatic hand injury.
Anesthesiology, 1979; 51: 565–566.

Sada T, Kobayashi T, Murakami S.
Continuous axillary brachial plexus block.
Can Anesth Soc J, 1983; 30: 201–205.

Sarnoff SJ, Sarnoff LC.
Prolonged peripheral nerve block by means of indwelling plastic catheter.
Treatment of hiccup. (Note on the electrical localization of peripheral nerve.)
Anesthesiology, 1951; 12: 270–275.

Sarton E, Olofsen E, Romberg R, et al.
Sex difference in morphine analgesia: an experimental study in healthy volunteers.
Anesthesiology, 2000; 93: 1245–1254.

Savoie FH, Field LD, Jenkins N, Mallon WJ, Phelps RA.
The pain control infusion pump for postoperative pain control in shoulder surgery.
Arthroscopy, 2000; 16: 339–342.

Sciard D, Matuszczak M, Gebhard R, Greger J, Al-Samsam T, Chelly JE.
Continuous lumbar plexus block for acute postoperative pain control in infants.
Anesthesiology, 2001; in press.

Selander D.
Catheter technique in axillary plexus block.
Acta Anaesth Scand, 1977; 21: 324–329.

Singelyn FJ, Gouverneur JM.
Postoperative analgesia after total hip arthroplasty: IV PCA with morphine, patient-controlled epidural analgesia, or continuous '3-in-1' block?: a prospective evaluation by our acute pain service in more than 1,300 patients.
J Clin Anesth, 1999; 11: 550–554.

Singelyn FJ, Aye F, Gouverneur JM.
Continuous popliteal nerve block: an original technique to provide postoperative analgesia after foot surgery.
Anesth Analg, 1997; 84: 383–386.

Singelyn FJ, Deyaert M, Joris D, Pendeville E, Gouverneur JM.
Effects of intravenous patient-controlled analgesia with morphine, continuous epidural analgesia, and continuous three-in-one block on postoperative pain and knee rehabilitation after unilateral total knee arthroplasty.
Anesth Analg, 1998; 87: 88–92.

Singelyn FJ, Seguy S, Gouverneur JM.
Interscalene brachial plexus analgesia after open shoulder surgery: continuous versus patient-controlled infusion.
Anesth Analg, 1999; 89: 1216–1220.

Singelyn FJ, Vanderelst PE, Gouverneur JM.
Extended femoral nerve sheath block after total hip arthroplasty: continuous versus patient-controlled techniques.
Anesth Analg, 2001; 92: 455–459.

Smith BE, Fischer HBJ, Scott PV.
Continuous sciatic nerve block.
Anesthesia, 1984; 39: 155–157.

Spansberg NM, Anker-Moller E, Dahl JB, Schultz P, Christensen EF.
The value of continuous blockade of the lumbar plexus as an adjunct to acetylsalicylic acid for pain relief after surgery for femoral neck fractures.
Eur J Anaesthesiol, 1996; 13: 410–412.

Stevens RD, Van Gessel E, Flory N, Fournier R, Gamulinz.
Lumbar plexus block reduces pain and blood loss associated with total hip arthroplasty.
Anesthesiology, 2000; 93: 115–121.

Stulberg BN, Insall JN, Williams GW, Ghelman B.
Deep-vein thrombosis following total knee replacement.
J Bone Joint Surgery, 1984; 64: 194–201.

Tobias JD.
Continuous femoral nerve block to provide analgesia following femur fracture in a paediatric ICU population.
Anaesth Intens Care, 1994; 22: 616–618.

Todd MM, Brown DL.
Regional anesthesia and postoperative pain management: long-term benefits from a short-term intervention.
Anesthesiology, 1999; 91: 1–2.

Tuominen M, Pitkanen M, Rosenberg PH.
Postoperative pain relief and bupivacaine plasma levels during continuous interscalene brachial plexus block.
Acta Anaesthesiol Scand, 1987; 31: 276–278.

Tuominen M, Haasio J, Hekali R, Rosenberg PH.
Continuous interscalene brachial plexus block: clinical efficacy, technical problems and bupivacaine plasma concentrations.
Acta Anaesthesiol Scand, 1989; 33: 84–88.

Vaghadia H, Kapnoudhis P, Jenkins LC, Taylor D.
Continuous lumbosacral block using a Tuohy needle and catheter technique.
Can J Anaesth, 1992; 39: 75–78.

2

EQUIPMENT AND DRUGS

CHAPTER
4

LOCAL ANESTHETICS

A. Casati

Introduction

Different local anesthetics are now available, including lidocaine (lignocaine), mepivacaine, prilocaine, etidocaine, bupivacaine, tetracaine (amethocaine), ropivacaine, and levobupivacaine. Each has preferential indications and contraindications, related mainly to their pharmacokinetic and pharmacodynamic properties.

In view of the need to limit the number of drugs in the formulary, we selected two short-acting local anesthetics of intermediate duration (lidocaine and mepivacaine) and two long-acting local anesthetics (bupivacaine and ropivacaine). More recently, levobupivacaine, a new long-acting local anesthetic, was also introduced into the market. Levobupivacaine is the pure left isomer of the racemic bupivacaine. Studies to evaluate the indications for levobupivacaine for continuous peripheral nerve blocks are in progress; preliminary data obtained in animals suggest that levobupivacaine has less systemic toxicity than racemic bupivacaine, and therefore may have the potential to substitute for the racemic formulation in the near future.

It is possible to optimize the advantages of each local anesthetic by combining them: a short-acting local anesthetic to reduce the onset time of the block, and a long-acting one to prolong the block for postoperative

analgesia. However, the ratio of advantages to disadvantages in this strategy requires further investigations, especially for continuous perineural infusions. On the other hand, for acute postoperative analgesia the use of low concentrations of local anesthetics enables a preferential sensory block to be induced, especially with ropivacaine, and so allows early active postoperative mobilization and rehabilitation.

Nerve roots anatomy and classification

The nerve roots are divided into three types according to their anatomic and functional properties: A fibers, B fibers, and C fibers. The efferent A fibers are responsible for motor impulses, and are divided into Aα, Aβ, and Aγ fibers. They are all myelinated, like the Aδ fibers, which are sensitive fibers that carry pressure and distension information. The B fibers are composed of the autonomic preganglionic fibers, while the C fibers include all the unmyelinated fibers of the posterior spinal roots, as well as the postganglionic autonomic fibers.

In the myelinated nerve roots, the action potential conduction proceeds from one Ranvier node to the other (jumping conduction). As the size of the fibers is proportional to the length between one Ranvier node and the next, the conduction speed of the action potential also increases with the size of the fibers. Generally, the larger the diameter of the nerve fibers the greater the amount of local anesthetic solution required to block the conduction. Thus, the smallest fibers are blocked sooner than are those with the largest diameters. The B fibers of the autonomic system constitute an exception to this rule: even though they are myelinated fibers, a low concentration of local anesthet-

Figure 4.1 ▶

Evolution of onset and recovery of nerve blockade in different types of nerve fibers.

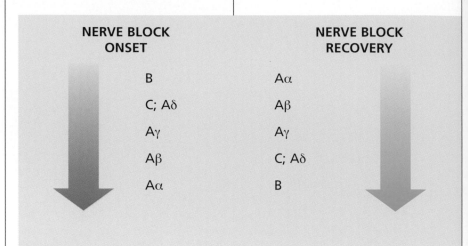

NERVE BLOCK ONSET	NERVE BLOCK RECOVERY
B	Aα
C; Aδ	Aβ
Aγ	Aγ
Aβ	C; Aδ
Aα	B

ic solution produces an effective blockade. This explains why the sympathetic blockade is observed before the block of the other fibers *(Figure 4.1)*.

It is possible to determine the minimum concentration of local anesthetic required to block only the small fibers, which are mainly responsible for nociception, with minimal or no block of the larger fibers. This produces good analgesia with minimal or no motor block, and is the basis of the differential sensory-motor blockade.

■ Chemical and physical properties

All local anesthetic molecules have an aromatic ring (structure 1 in *Figure 4.2*) and one aminotype portion (structure 4 in *Figure 4.2*) which are bound together by either an ester or amido link (structure 2 in *Figure 4.2*). Accordingly, we can identify two different groups: aminoester local anesthetics, like procaine, or the aminoamide local anesthetics, like lidocaine *(Figure 4.3)*.

The aromatic ring is responsible for the lipophilic properties of the molecule, which are directly related to its potency, whereas the amino portion at the other end of the molecule is responsible for its hydrophilic properties, which affect its diffusibility and ability to penetrate the nerve fibers. The type of link between structures 1 and 4 influences the resistance to hydrolysis of the molecule: the aminoamide local anesthetics are more resistant than the aminoester ones, which results in a longer duration of action.

Different hypotheses have been suggested to explain the mechanisms of local anesthetics; however, it seems that all local anesthetics produce structural changes in the cell membrane that affect the function of voltage-dependent ionic channels, which are activated by depolarization. This increases the activation threshold of the action potential, and reduces the propagation of the action potential itself along the nerve fibers, resulting in a complete block of the nerve fiber function. Table 4.1 shows the main chemophysical properties of the anesthetic drugs discussed here, as well as their reported equipotent concentrations.

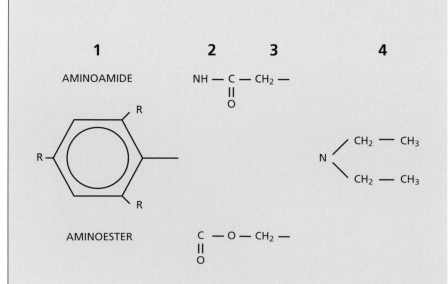

Different structural units of local anesthetics.

◀ **Figure 4.2**

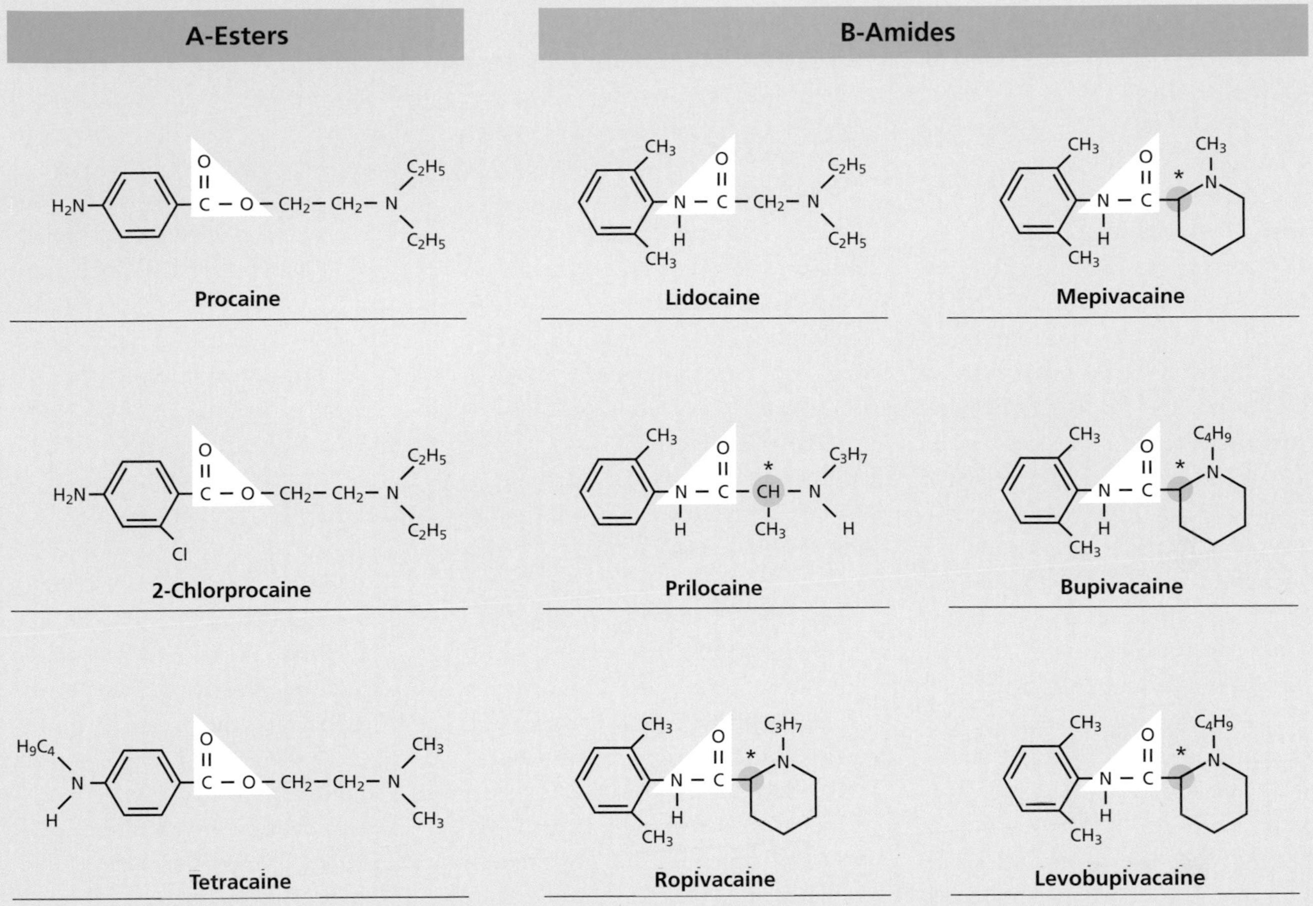

A-Esters	B-Amides	

Procaine

Lidocaine

Mepivacaine

2-Chlorprocaine

Prilocaine

Bupivacaine

Tetracaine

Ropivacaine

Levobupivacaine

▲ Figure 4.3

Local anesthetic structures with the ester and amide link shown within the superimposed triangle. When present, the asymmetric carbon is circled, shaded and marked with an *. (Adapted from Di Fazio et al. 2000, with permission from Mosby.)

Table 4.1   Chemical and physical properties of the main anesthetics, including reported equipotent concentrations

Property	Lidocaine	Mepivacaine	Bupivacaine	Ropivacaine	Levobupivacaine
Molecular weight	234	246	288	274	288
pK_a	7.7	7.6	8.1	8.1	8.1
Liposolubility	4	1	30	2.8	30
Partition coefficient	2.9	0.8	28	9	28
Protein binding (%)	65	75	95	94	95
Equipotent concentration (%)	2	1.5	0.5	0.75	0.5

Adapted from Di Fazio et al. 2000, with permission from Mosby.

Clinical properties

The choice of local anesthetic for peripheral nerve blocks is based mainly on the onset time and duration of the block, as well as on the ability to produce a differential sensory motor block and on the safety margin. The onset time of local anesthetics is influenced by the molecule's pK_a (the higher the pK_a the slower the onset time of the nerve block in a physiological environment) and diffusibility.

On the other hand, the ability to cross the cell membrane depends on the molecular weight and the liposolubility of the molecule. All local anesthetics have nearly the same molecular weight, but the diffusibility of the local anesthetic molecule from the injection site depends on its hydrophilic properties. The non-ionized form of the molecule is more soluble in lipids than the ionized form, so it can cross the cell membrane more easily, but it diffuses less easily. The commercial solutions of local anesthetics have an acidic pH, while the pK_a of the different local anesthetics ranges from 7.9 to 8.1. Accordingly, the ionized form, which is less lipophilic, is present in a greater proportion than the non-ionized form.

To shorten the onset time it is possible to increase the dose, volume, or concentration of a given local anesthetic (Covino and Bush 1975, Vester-Andresen et al. 1982, 1984, Casati et al. 1998, 1999, Fanelli et al. 1998).

Other strategies include modification of the pK_a of the anesthetic solution by warming it or adding sodium bicarbonate to increase the number of non-ionized local anesthetic molecules (Coventry and Todd 1989, Capogna et al. 1995), especially with either lidocaine or mepivacaine. It is more difficult to alkalinize ropivacaine, bupivacaine, or levobupivacaine, because of their high pK_a (Coventry and Todd 1989).

Another important aspect that deserves consideration is the pH of tissues: for example, local tissue acidosis related to inflammation can increase the ionized form of local anesthetic, reducing its effectiveness (Bennett 1984).

The potency of a local anesthetic is usually evaluated by the minimum effective concentration (C_m), the minimum anesthetic concentration that, within 5 minutes, reduces by 50% the action potential of a nerve fiber bathed in a solution of pH 7.2–7.4 and stimulated by a 30 Hz current (Gallo et al. 1992).

The potency of local anesthetics is strictly related to their lipid solubility: the more lipid soluble a local anesthetic is the greater the potency, and consequently the lower its C_m.

The minimum effective concentration of a local anesthetic also changes according to the diameter of the nerve fiber (Covino 1986, Butterworth and Strichartz 1990, Richards and McConachie 1995). While the total amount of local anesthetic affects the onset, degree, and duration of the nerve block, its concentration influences the intensity of the blockade.

The smallest fibers (Aδ, B, and C), with a slower conduction speed, are more sensitive to the blocking activity of the local anesthetic solution than are those with a larger diameter (Aβ and Aα), with fast conduction. In other words, the smallest fibers need a lower C_m than those of larger size. This aspect is related to the number of anesthetic molecules available to block the conduction: when using low concentrations the small number of local anesthetic molecules available blocks only the small fibers (Covino 1986, Butterworth and Strichartz 1990, Richards and McConachie 1995). A possible explanation is the need to block three consecutive Ranvier nodes to produce a complete nerve block. Since the distance between consecutive Ranvier nodes increases as the diameter of the nerve fiber increases, low concentrations of local anesthetic block three consecutive Ranvier nodes only in the small nerve fibers, and not in the large ones. This is the basis of the differential sensory-motor blockade, which is more evident with lipophilic agents of high pK_a, such as bupivacaine, ropivacaine, and, probably, levobupivacaine.

Both protein binding and elimination from the site of injection influence the duration of action of local anesthetic solutions (Scott et al 1972, Covino 1986, Butter worth and Strichartz 1990, Richards and McConachie 1995).

Additives

Different additives can be used with local anesthetics to modify the clinical properties and potentiate and/or modify the pharmacology and/or pharmacokinetic properties.

The additives most frequently used in clinical practice include the vasoactive drugs, alkalinization, clonidine, and opioids.

Vasoconstrictors

The duration of a local anesthetic depends on the duration of the contact between the local anesthetic agent and the nerve fibers as well as on the number of local anesthetic molecules that act on the nerve fibers themselves. To produce a more intense and longer lasting block the dose of local anesthetic solution can be increased (changing the volume and/or concentration), or the amount of local anesthetic removed for units of time from the receptor site can be reduced. Epinephrine (adrenaline), in a dose of 5 µg/ml (1:200,000), reduces the vascular absorption of local anesthetics, increasing their concentration at the target site.

This provides a clinically significant prolongation of the blocks (Covino 1986, Butterworth and Strichartz 1990, Richards and McConachie 1995). Adding epinephrine to solutions of lidocaine, mepivacaine, or bupivacaine used for upper extremity peripheral blocks increases the duration and the intensity of the block. However, adding epinephrine to ropivacaine does not result in clinically relevant effects on the duration of the block. This could in part arise from intrinsic vasoconstrictive properties.

Furthermore, adding a vasoconstrictor can reduce the perfusion of the vasa nervorum, which potentially increases the risk of an ischemic nerve injury. For these reasons the extensive use of epinephrine as an adjuvant to local anesthetic solutions for continuous peripheral nerve blocks is not recommended, especially if continuous infusion rather than an intermittent bolus technique is used to manage postoperative pain.

Alkalinization

The pH of commercially available solutions of local anesthetic ranges from 3 to 6.5 and the pK_a ranges from 7.6 to 8.9. Solutions containing epinephrine are even more acidic than are those without it. As mentioned above, alkalinization of local anesthetic solutions can reduce the onset time of a nerve block induced with lidocaine or mepivacaine. Alkalinization is usually obtained by adding 1 meq/l of sodium bicarbonate to 10 ml of lidocaine 2%, mepivacaine 2%, and chlorprocaine 3%; different results have been reported when sodium bicarbonate is added to bupivacaine (Coventry and Todd 1989, Di Fazio 1991, Capogna et al. 1995, Tezlaff et al. 1995). However, even though changing the pH of the anesthetic solution may shorten the onset time of the block, there are no clinically relevant advantages when a continuous peripheral nerve block is used. Finally, the stability of the anesthetic solution with bicarbonate is unknown. As this remains in the infusion bag for up to 24 hours before being renewed, we do not recommend that sodium bicarbonate be used for continuous peripheral nerve blocks.

Alpha-2-agonists

The analgesic effects of alpha-2-agonists are well known, and clonidine is widely used for chronic and acute pain management. Clonidine has been shown to inhibit the action potential of Aα and C fibers in desheathed sciatic nerves, while alpha-2-adrenergic receptors activated by clonidine have been demonstrated at primary afferent terminals, on neurons in the super-ficial laminae of the spinal cord, and in brainstem nuclei, which are involved in analgesia. The inhibition of norepinephrine (noradrenaline) release, mediated by clonidine interaction with alpha-2-adrenergic presynaptic receptors, could be an alternative explanation for the enhancing effect of the peripheral administration of clonidine. Also, the peripheral antinociception induced by clonidine has been related to the local release of an enkephalin-like substance mediated by alpha-2-adrenoceptors (Khasar et al. 1995, Bernard and Macaire 1997). The addition of clonidine to local anesthetic solutions is known to improve peripheral nerve blocks; it reduces the onset time, prolongs postoperative analgesia, and improves the efficacy of nerve block during surgery (Maze and Tranquilli 1991, Salonen et al. 1992, Khasar et al. 1995, Bernard and Macaire 1997, Casati et al. 2000, 2001b). The addition of low doses of clonidine is also used for continuous peripheral nerve blocks, at a concentration as low as 1 µg/ml (Singelyn et al. 1997, 1999, 2001, Capdevila et al. 1999). The rationale for adding clonidine is to minimize the doses of local anesthetic solution required to produce an effective postoperative analgesia, and thus reduce the risks of local anesthetic-related side effects. However, even though the use of clonidine at these doses and concentrations seems reasonably effective and safe, randomized, prospective trials are still needed to evaluate its efficacy for continuous peripheral nerve blocks.

Opioids

Opioids are known to exert their analgesic activity directly in the central nervous system (CNS), and the addition of opioids to local anesthetic solutions improves the quality of anesthesia and postoperative analgesia during epidural and subarachnoid block (Chrubasik et al. 1993). An improvement in the onset time, quality, and duration of nerve blocks has also been reported by adding opioids to local anesthetic solutions for peripheral nerve blockades (Racz et al. 1982). In fact, opioid receptors have been demonstrated on primary afferent neurons and their expression is increased by inflammation (Fields et al. 1980). Nonetheless, other studies have failed to demonstrate clinically relevant advantages from adding opioids to local anesthetic solutions for peripheral nerve blocks (Flecther et al. 1994, Magistris et al. 2000, Fanelli et al. 2001).

Some authors also reported data on the use of small concentrations of opioids for continuous peripheral nerve blocks, claiming positive results after the use of either 0.1 μg/ml sufentanil (Singelyn et al. 1999, 2001) or 0.03 mg/ml morphine (Capdevila et al. 1999). Further controlled, randomized trials are required to evaluate the efficacy of small concentrations of opioids for continuous peripheral nerve blocks.

■ Toxicity

All anesthetic drugs can generate allergic reactions, which are mainly related to the use of aminoester drugs, like procaine. The haptenic reaction is related to para-aminoben-

8. Cardiac arrest

7. Respiratory arrest

6. Coma

5. Seizures

4. Muscular spasm

3. Tinnitus, auditory hallucinations

2. Paresthesias in the mouth and tongue

1. Drowsiness

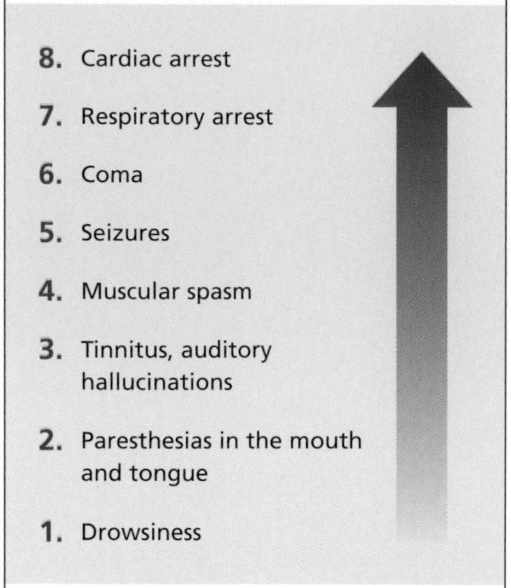

▲ **Figure 4.4**

Systemic toxicity related to local anesthetic.

zoic acid. When using amide anesthetic solutions the incidence of these adverse effects is much lower, and mainly associated with antibacterial additives similar to para-aminobenzoic acid, used mainly in multidose ampules.

Rarely, local toxic reactions are also observed. These adverse effects are rare when using clinically relevant concentrations of the anesthetic solution, but can lead to severe and permanent complications in cases of an intraneural injection. For this reason the block should always be placed in an awake (though slightly sedated) and co-operative patient, to maintain his or her protective escape response in case of an unwanted intraneural injection.

Systemic toxic reactions can be observed with overdosing, such as when combined blocks are used, or with an unwanted intravascular injection: the severity of these systemic reactions is related to the maximum plasma concentration achieved.

Systemic toxicity related to local anesthetics *(Figure 4.4)* arises from the depressant effects on all excitatory tissues, including the CNS and heart. The toxic potential of a local anesthetic is strictly associated with its lipophilic properties: bupivacaine is the most lipophilic aminoamide molecule and it is also the most toxic.

Clinical research has shown that left isomers of local anesthetic solutions are associated with lower cardiovascular toxicity than right isomers. Indeed, ropivacaine is less cardiotoxic than racemic bupivacaine, even though its lower lipid solubility accounts for a slightly reduced potency (Capogna et al. 1999). Interestingly, recent animal studies demonstrated that ropivacaine is less toxic than bupivacaine at both equivalent and equipotent doses (Dony et al. 2000). While the use of similar doses and concentrations of either ropivacaine or bupivacaine at anesthetic concentrations (≥0.5%) results in similar clinical effects (Casati et al. 2001a), the reduced potency of ropivacaine is more evident at the low concentrations used for postoperative pain relief. For this reason 0.2% concentrations of ropivacaine are usually used for postoperative analgesia, with clinical effects similar to those produced by bupivacaine 0.15%.

Levobupivacaine is the pure left isomer of bupivacaine, and seems associated with fewer toxic effects than the racemic formulation (Huang et al. 1998).

The depressant effect on the cardiovascular function is undoubtedly the most dangerous complication of local anesthetic administration: this depressant effect is the result of the direct negative inotropic and chronotropic effects associated with severe alterations of heart function.

The mechanism of action is not completely understood, but it is probably related to a profound interference with the metabolism of heart myocytes. This is also linked to a significant alteration of the calcium metabolism in the heart muscle, because of the reduction of energy production in the mitochondria (Sztark et al. 1998). Usually, the cardiovascular effects occur with doses 2–4 times higher than those that produce CNS complications (Denson and Mazoit 1991). Ropivacaine is associated with depressant effects that are four times lower than those of bupivacaine. Further, the negative effects are more likely to be reversible than those produced by bupivacaine, because of the prolonged binding of bupivacaine to the heart.

Accordingly, low concentrations of ropivacaine are preferable to bupivacaine for continuous peripheral nerve blocks.

The toxic reactions induced by local anesthetics can occur immediately after injection (intravascular injection) or can be delayed for 30–45 minutes after injection (systemic absorption from the injection site). For this reason, patients who receive a local anesthetic injection should be monitored carefully for at least 1 hour, and the injection should always be performed slowly with repeated aspirations every 5 ml to exclude the intravascular injection.

■ Clinical use

The choice of anesthetic solution must be tailored to the patient's characteristics as well as to the safe dose for the type of block and effect (anesthesia versus analgesia) sought. With a continuous perineural technique, a block is best achieved by using a short-onset, intermediate-duration anesthetic solution like mepivacaine or lidocaine at concentrations between 1.5% and 2% (reducing the concentration allows the use of larger volumes without the risk of overdosing). Some authors use combinations of anesthetic solutions with different kinetic properties: the most frequently used mixture is a combination of a short-onset anesthetic, like mepivacaine, with a long-duration anesthetic, like bupivacaine or ropivacaine. From a toxicological standpoint, these mixtures do not seem to reduce the overall toxicity, since the free concentration of the most toxic anesthetic is similar to that produced by using it alone in the same volume, because of competitive binding to the protein carriers between the two anesthetic drugs (Denson and Mazoit 1991). The volumes and doses of local anesthetic depend on the type of surgery (e.g., single block or combination of different blocks, as for the lower limb) and the use of sedation or light general anesthesia during surgery (specific therapeutic schemes are provided for the technique). Always consider the maximum doses suggested for each anesthetic drug (Table 4.2).

Postoperative analgesia

From a theoretical standpoint, we can either use an anesthetic of short onset and duration, or a long-acting one. The use of a short-acting anesthetic, such as lidocaine, allows the possibility of a fast recovery of normal neuronal function after the infusion is stopped, which enables an easier neurological evaluation (Capdevila et al. 1998, 1999). However, most authors prefer long-acting local anesthetics, like bupivacaine or ropivacaine. Recently, Borgeat et al. (2001) demonstrated

Table 4.2	Block characteristics, concentrations, and doses suggested to induce a peripheral nerve block				
Anesthetic	Concentration (%)	Onset	Duration (h)	Maximum dose (mg)	pH
Lidocaine	1.5–2	fast	1–2	300 500 + epinephrine	6.5
Mepivacaine	1.5–2	fast	2–3	500 600 + epinephrine	4.5
Bupivacaine	0.5	slow	4–12	150 225 + epinephrine	4.5–6
Ropivacaine	0.75	slow	2–6	225–300	4–6

that ropivacaine 0.2% induced preferential sensory block, with a minimal motor block.

The continuous administration of local anesthetic solution can be based on an intermittent bolus technique or the use of infusion devices. Infusion devices (Chapter 5) can provide continuous infusion at a rate between 5 and 10 ml/h, or provide patient-controlled analgesia, which allows optimization of the analgesic efficacy and minimizes the total amount of anesthetic drug used (Singelyn et al. 1999, 2001, Borgeat et al. 2000, Singelyn and Gouverneur 2000, Di Benedetto et al. 2002).

Table 4.3 shows the concentrations and regimens, as well as the concentrations of additives, suggested for continuous peripheral nerve blocks with the main anesthetic solutions described in the literature and used in our clinical experience.

Table 4.3 Concentrations and infusion rates suggested for continuous peripheral nerve blocks

Anesthetic	Concentration (%)	Infusion rate (ml/h)	Additives
Lidocaine	1	6–10	Clonidine, 1 µg/ml and/or morphine, 0.03 mg/ml
Bupivacaine	0.125–0.25	6–10	Clonidine, 1 µg/ml and/or sufentanil, 0.1 µg/ml
Ropivacaine	0.15–0.2	6–10	Clonidine, 1 µg/ml and/or sufentanil, 0.1 µg/ml

CHAPTER

5 EQUIPMENT

J.E. Chelly

Introduction

The success of continuous perineural infusion techniques for the postoperative management of pain in orthopedic patients depends as much on the appropriate technical skills of the anesthesiologist's placement of the catheter as on the appropriate choice of material. Today, except for the placement of iliofascial and psoas compartment catheters, the use of a nerve stimulator has become standard. Furthermore, several companies provide catheter sets with material necessary to secure these catheters as well as infusion pumps for inpatients and ambulatory patients.

Catheters

The development of different catheter sets is based on a choice between:
- type of introducer, either plastic catheter or insulated needle; and
- type of catheter, which may depend on the technique used to place the catheter (catheters with or without a stylet, Seldinger technique, stimulating catheters).

Since the first introduction of the continuous perineural technique, the material used has evolved significantly, but always around the same basic principles. As early as 1951 the concept of using an introducer

Table 5.1 Approach and needles used

Approach	Type of needle	Length (cm)	Direction of the bevel
Interscalene			
Tangential	Straight needle	3.5–5.0	To the axilla
Winnie	Tuohy	3.5	To the axilla
Supraclavicular	Tuohy	3.5–5.0	Upward
Infraclavicular			
Vertical	Tuohy	5.0	To the axilla
Raj	Tuohy	10.0–15.0	Upward
Axillary			
30°	Tuohy	5.0	Upward
Tangential	Straight needle	5.0	
Sciatic			
Parasacral	Tuohy	10.0	Lateral
Gluteal	Tuohy	10.0	Cephalad
Anterior	Tuohy	15.0	Cephalad
Lateral popliteal	Tuohy	10.0	Cephalad
Posterior popliteal	Tuohy	10.0	Cephalad
Lumbar plexus/femoral			
Lumbar plexus	Tuohy	10.0	Cephalad
Femoral	Tuohy	5.0	Cephalad and upward

needle followed by the placement of tubing and its contained stylet was described. Sarnoff and Sarnoff (1951) reported the use of an 18-gauge introducer and polyethylene tubing and its contained stylet needle. The authors also described the electrical stimulation of the stylet to verify the proper positioning of the needle.

It took almost 50 years for companies to market a stimulating catheter. In the 1970s, epidural sets were used for the placement of catheters in the psoas compartment (Brands and Callanan 1978), while

the use of a Teflon indwelling catheter needle (introducing catheter) was reported for the placement of an axillary catheter (Manriquez and Pallares 1978).

In the past few years, the quality of the catheters has improved. In 1996, Hirst reported the use of an 18-gauge insulated Tuohy introducer. The insulated Tuohy needle has become the preferred choice for many anesthesiologists *(Table 5.1)*.

Introducer plastic catheter. These are 15- to 17-gauge plastic catheters with a contained metallic guide. These introducer catheters are in various lengths from 50 mm to 150 mm depending on the indications and the manufacturer *(Figure 5.1)*. The metallic guide is connected to a nerve stimulator and removed once the plastic introducer catheter is properly positioned.

Although Selander (1977) recommended the use of an introducer plastic catheter for perineural infusions of local anesthetic, an epidural catheter is usually placed through the plastic introducer catheter.

Insulated introducer needles. The use of introducer needles has grown significantly in the past few years. Although various types of needle have been proposed, including b-beveled and Sprotte needles, the insulated Tuohy needle *(Figure 5.2)* has become the preferred choice, as it represents the best compromise between the advantages and disadvantages of other needles.

Indeed, the insulated Tuohy needle allows partial control of the direction of the catheter by orientation of the bevel. Further, the tip of the Tuohy needle enables the catheter to exit the needle at an angle closer to the angle between the needle and the nerve that needs to be blocked.

In fact, except for a few specific approaches described for the placement of catheters only (such as the axillary and tangential interscalene approaches), the nerve is approached at an angle from between 30 and 45° (femoral, interscalene) to 90° (lumbar plexus, lateral sciatic) using the same technique as for a single injection.

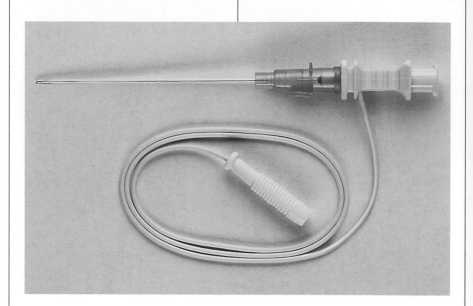

▲ **Figure 5.1**

Plastic introducer catheter with stimulating guide.

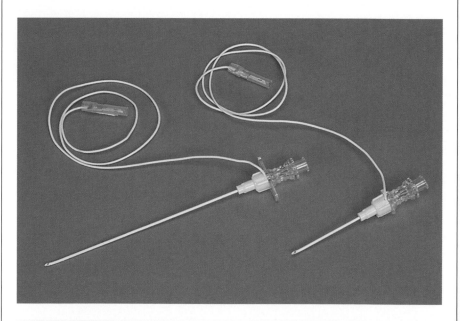

▲ **Figure 5.2**

Stimulating Tuohy needle introducer.

Although the use of a straight needle is appropriate for techniques approaching the nerve tangentially, this type of needle does not allow the anesthesiologist to properly direct the catheter when the nerve is approached obliquely or perpendicularly.

Type of catheters

There are basically four types of catheters for continuous peripheral nerve blocks:

- 20-gauge epidural catheter *(Figure 5.3)*;
- 20- or 21-gauge epidural catheter

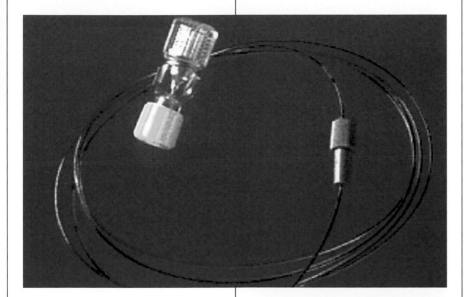

20-gauge epidural catheter.

Recently, some companies have introduced specific devices to fix the catheter at the skin with adhesive tapes, on which the catheter is locked. Again, no clinical evidence supports the use of one specific device rather than another to secure the catheter to the skin; however, accurate catheter fixation is a critical factor to maximize the success rate and prevent postoperative displacement of the catheter.

with metallic stylet *(Figure 5.4)*;
* 20-gauge catheter to be threaded over a wire using the Seldinger technique *(Figure 5.5)*; and
* stimulating catheter (21-gauge catheter with a metallic stylet that allows stimulation).

As yet no clear evidence supports one specific type of catheter, especially if the catheter is not advanced more than 3–4 cm from the tip of the needle.

The stimulating catheter appears interesting, but an appropriate evaluation of the cost–benefit ratio needs to be conducted to determine the advantage of each type. In Europe, all catheters are connected to bacterial filters.

Catheter fixation

Our perineural catheters are secured in place with 12 mm x 100 mm Stery-Strips (3M Health Care, St Paul, MN, USA) and covered with a transparent Tegaderm (3M Health Care, St Paul, MN, USA). The transparent dressing allows control at the insertion site of the catheter during the postoperative evaluations.

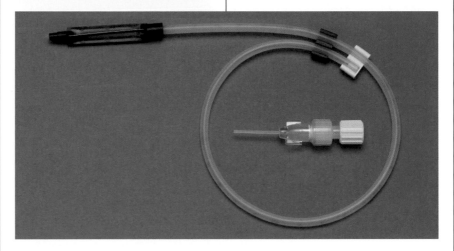

▲ Figure 5.4

20- or 21-gauge catheter with metallic stylet.

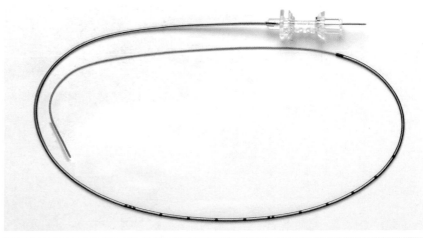

▲ Figure 5.5

20-gauge introducer for the Seldinger technique.

■ Infusion pumps

Inpatient pumps

The pumps used for postoperative perineural infusions need to satisfy certain criteria, including a light weight to allow early mobilization, the use of a wide range of infusion rates, and patient-controlled analgesia. In addition, the pump should have some safety features built in, including stopping whenever the protective box is opened or if high pressures are encountered in the infusion system *(Figure 5.6)*.

Outpatient pumps

At present there are two types of ambulatory pumps:
- elastomeric or electronic pumps, which provide a constant infusion rate only (2, 5, or 10 ml/h, or higher; *Figure 5.7*); and
- patient-controlled analgesia (PCA) electronic pumps that not only allow control of the basal rate, but also provide additional boluses with variable lockout times *(Figure 5.8)*.

For ambulatory orthopedic indications we prefer the use of PCA pumps, which provide the opportunity to minimize and tailor the amount of local anesthetics required, with safe, effective, and long-lasting pain control.

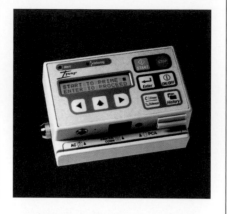

▲ **Figure 5.6**

Example of eletronic pump for patient-controlled analgesia (PCA).

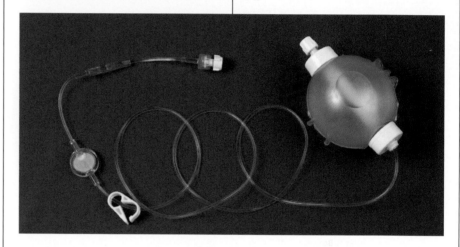

▲ **Figure 5.7**

Example of a disposable elastomeric pump with constant infusion rate.

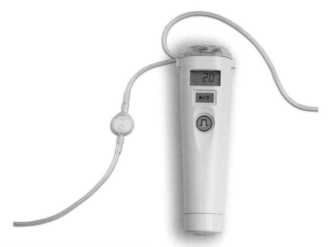

▲ **Figure 5.8**

Example of an electronic PCA pump for outpatient infusion.

References

Bennett CR.
*Monheim's Local anesthesia
and pain control in dental practice.*
Mosby, 7th ed, 1984.

Bernard JM, Macaire P.
*Dose-range effects of clonidine added
to lidocaine for brachial plexus block.*
Anesthesiology, 1997; 87: 277-284.

Borgeat A, Perschak H, Bird P, Hodler J.
*Patient-controlled interscalene analgesia
with ropivacaine 0.2% versus patient-
controlled intravenous analgesia after
major shoulder surgery: effects on
diaphragmatic and respiratory function.*
Anesthesiology, 2000; 92: 102-108.

**Borgeat A, Kalberer F, Jacob H, Ruetsch YA,
Gerber C.**
*Patient-controlled interscalene analgesia
with ropivacaine 0.2% versus bupivacaine
0.15% after major open shoulder surgery:
the effects on hand motor function..*
Anesth Analg, 2001; 92: 218-213.

Brands E, Callanan VI.
*Continuous lumbar plexus block – analgesia
for femoral neck fractures.*
Anesth Intens Care, 1978; 6: 256-258.

Butterworth J, Strichartz G.
*Molecular mechanisms of local
anesthesia: A review.*
Anesth Analg, 1990; 72: 711-734.

**Capdevilla X, Biboulet P, Bouregba M,
Rubenovitch J, Jaber S.**
*Bilateral continuous 3-in-1 nerve
blockade for postoperative pain relief
after bilateral femoral shaft surgery.*
J Clin Anesth, 1998; 10: 606-609.

**Capdevilla X, Barthelet Y, Biboulet P,
Ryckwaert Y, Rubenovitch J, d'Athis F.**
*Effects of perioperative analgesic technique
on the surgical outcome and duration
of rehabilitation after major knee surgery.*
Anesthesiology, 1999; 91: 8-15.

**Capogna G, Celleno D, Laudano D,
Giunta F.**
*Alkalinization of local anesthetics.
Which block, which local anesthetic?*
Reg Anesth, 1995; 20: 369-377.

Capogna G, Celleno D, Fusco P, et al.
*Relative potencies of bupivacaine
and ropivacaine for analgesia in labour.*
Br J Anaesth, 1999; 82: 371-373.

**Casati A, Leoni A, Aldegheri G,
Berti M, Torri G, Fanelli G.**
*A double-blind study of axillary
brachial plexus block by 0.75%
ropivacaine or 2% mepivacaine.*
Eur J Anaesth, 1998; 15: 549-552.

Casati A, Fanelli G, Borghi B, Torri G.
*A randomized blind evaluation
of either 0.5%, 0.75%, 1% ropivacaine
or 2% mepivacaine for lower limb
peripheral nerve blocks.*
Anesthesiology, 1999; 90: 1047-1053.

Casati A, Magistris L, Fanelli G, et al.
*Small dose clonidine prolongs postoperative
analgesia after sciatic-femoral nerve block
with 0.75% ropivacaine for foot surgery.*
Anesth Analg, 2000; 91: 388-392.

**Casati A, Fanelli G, Magistris L, Beccaria P,
Berti M, Torri G.**
*Minimum local anesthetic volume blocking
the femoral nerve in 50% of cases.
A double blind comparison between 0.5%
ropivacaine and 0.5% bupivacaine.*
Anesth Analg, 2001a; 92: 205-208.

**Casati A, Magistris L, Beccaria P, Cappelleri
G, Aldegheri G, Torri G.**
*Improving postoperative analgesia after
axillary brachial plexus anesthesia with
0.75% ropivacaine: a double-blind
evaluation of adding clonidine. Minerva
Anestesiol, 2001b; 67: 407-412.*

Chrubasik J, Chrubasik S, Mather L.
Postoperative epidural opioids.
Springer-Verlag, 1993.

Coventry DM, Todd JG.
*Alkalinization of bupivacaine for sciatic
nerve blockade.*
Anaesthesia, 1989; 44: 467-470.

Covino BG.
Pharmacology of local anaesthetic agents.
Br J Anaesth, 1986; 58: 701-716.

Covino BG, Bush DF.
Clinical evaluation of local anaesthetic agents.
Br J Anaesth, 1975; 47: 289-296.

Denson DD, Mazoit JX.
*Physiology, pharmacology and toxicity of
local anesthetics: adult and pediatric
considerations. In: Raj PP. Clinical practice
of regional anesthesia.*
Churchill-Livingstone, 1991, pp. 73-105.

Di Benedetto P, Casati A, Bertini L.
*Continuous subgluteus sciatic nerve block
after orthopedic foot and ankle surgery:
comparison of two infusion techniques.*
Reg Anesth Pain Med 2002; in press.

Di Fazio CA.
*Adjuvant techniques to success
in regional anesthesia. In: Raj PP. Clinical
practice of regional anesthesia.*
Churchill-Livingstone, 1991, pp. 73-105.

Di Fazio CA, Woods AM Rowlingson JC.
*Drugs commonly used for nerve blocking:
pharmacology of local anesthetics. In: Raj
PP; editor.
Practical management of pain, 3rd ed.,*
Mosby, 2000.

Dony P, Dewinde V, Vanderick B, et al.
*The comparative toxicity of ropivacaine
and bupivacaine at equipotent doses in rats.*
Anesth Analg, 2000; 91: 1489-1492.

Fanelli G, Casati A, Beccaria P, et al.
*A double-blind comparison of ropivacaine,
bupivacaine and mepivacaine during sciatic
and femoral nerve blockade.*
Anesth Analg, 1998; 87: 597-600.

Fanelli G, Casati A, Magistris M, et al.
*Fentanyl does not improve the nerve block
characteristics of axillary brachial plexus
anaesthesia performed with ropivacaine.*
Acta Anaesthesiol Scand, 2001;
45: 590-594.

Fields HL, Emcen PC, Leigh BK, et al.
*Multiple opiate receptor sites on primary
afferent fibres.*
Nature, 1980; 284: 351-353.

Flecther D, Kuhlman G, Samii K.
*Addition of fentanyl to 1.5% lidocaine does
not increase the success of axillary plexus
block.*
Reg Anesth, 1994; 19: 183-188.

Gallo F, Giusti P, Alberti S, Valenti S.
Farmacologia degli anestetici locali.
ALR 1, 1992; 2: 80-92.

**Hirst GC, Lang SA, Dust WN,
Cassidy JD, Yip RW.**
*Femoral nerve block. Single injection
versus continuous infusion
for total knee arthroplasty.*
Reg Anesth, 1996; 21: 292-297.

**Huang Y, Pryor ME, Mather LE,
Veering BT.**
*Cardiovascular and central nervous system
effects of intravenous levobupivacaine
and bupivacaine in sheep.*
Anesth Analg, 1998; 86: 797-804.

Khasar SG, Green PG, Chou B, Levine JD.
*Peripheral nociceptive effects of alpha2-
adrenergic receptor agonist in the rat.*
Neuroscience, 1995; 66: 427-432.

Magistris L, Casati A, Albertin A, et al.
*Combined sciatic-femoral nerve block
with 0.75% ropivacaine: effects of adding
a systemically inactive dose of fentanyl.
Eur J Anaesthesiol, 2000; 17: 348-353.*

Manriquez RG, Pallares V.
*Continuous brachial plexus block
for prolonged sympathectomy
and control of pain.
Anesth Analg, 1978; 57: 128-130.*

Maze M, Tranquilli W.
*Alpha-2 adrenoreceptor agonists:
defining the role in clinical anesthesia.
Anesthesiology, 1991; 74: 581-605.*

Racz H, Gunning K, Della Santa.
*Evaluation on the of the effect of perineural
morphyne on the quality post operative
analgesia after axillary plexus block.
Acta Anaesthesiol Scand, 1982;
26: 519-523.*

Richards A, McConachie I.
*The pharmacology of local anesthetic drugs.
Curr Anaesth Critical Care, 1995; 6: 41-47.*

Salonen MA, Kanto JH, Maze M.
*Clinical interactions with alpha-2
adrenergic agonists in anesthetic practice.
J Clin Anesth 1992; 4:164-172.*

Sarnoff SJ, Sarnoff LC.
*Prolonged peripheral nerve block by means
of indwelling plastic catheter. Treatment
of hiccup. (Note on the electrical localization
of peripheral nerve.)
Anesthesiology, 1951; 12: 270-275.*

Scott DB, Jebson PJ, Braid DP,
Orengren B, Frisch P.
*Factors affecting plasma level
of lidocaine and prilocaine.
Br J Anesth, 1972; 44: 1040-1048.*

Selander D.
*Catheter technique in axillary block.
Acta Anaesth Scand, 1977; 21: 324-329.*

Singelyn FJ, Gouverneur JM.
*Extended "three-in-one" block after total
knee arthroplasty: continuous versus
patient-controlled techniques.
Anesth Analg, 2000; 91: 176-180.*

Singelyn FJ, Aye F, Gouverneur JM.
*Continuous popliteal sciatic nerve block:
an original technique to provide
postoperative analgesia after foot surgery.
Anesth Analg, 1997; 84: 383-386.*

Singelyn FJ, Seguy S, Gouverneur JM.
*Interscalene brachial plexus analgesia after
open shoulder surgery: continuous versus
patient-controlled infusion.
Anesth Analg, 1999; 89: 1216-1220.*

Singelyn FJ, Vanderelst PE,
Gouverneur JM.
*Extended femoral nerve sheath block
after total hip arthroplasty: continuous
versus patient-controlled techniques.
Anesth Analg, 2001; 92: 455-459.*

Sztark F, Malgat M, Dabade P, Mazat JP.
*Comparison of the effects of bupivacaine
and ropivacaine on heart cell mitocondrial
bioenergetics.
Anesthesiology, 1998; 88: 1340-1349.*

Tezlaff J, Yoon H, Brems J, Javorsky T.
*Alkalinization of mepivacaine improveses
the quality of motor block associated
with interscalene brachial plexus
anesthesia for shoulder surgery.
Reg Anesth, 1995; 20: 128-132.*

Vester-Andersen T, Christiansen C,
Sørensen M, Eriksen C.
*Perivascular axillary block I:
Blockade following 40 mL of 1%
mepivacaine with adrenaline.
Acta Anaesthesiol Scand, 1982;
26: 519-523.*

Vester-Andersen T, Husum B, Lindeburg T,
Borrits L, Gøthgen I.
*Perivascular axillary block IV:
Blockade following 40, 50 or 60 mL
of mepivacaine 1% with adrenaline.
Acta Anaesthesiol Scand, 1984; 28: 99-105.*

3

TECHNIQUES

READY TO START

A. Casati, J.E. Chelly

Continuous peripheral nerve blocks have become an important and effective approach for pain treatment in orthopedic patients; however, these techniques are more effective when included in a multidisciplinary and multimodal approach to the patient's pain management.

All specialists, including surgeons, anesthesiologists, recovery and ward nurses, physical therapists, and pharmacists, who care for patients must work together throughout the perioperative period to improve the patient's well-being and outcome.

Preoperative communication and interaction enable the optimum timing and most appropriate strategy for anesthesia and acute postoperative management to be chosen according to the condition of the patient and the surgical and postoperative physical therapy requirements.

Interaction and communication with the pharmacist and nursing staff facilitate both a timely start of the acute postoperative pain treatment and immediate rehabilitation. Different patients and surgery require a combination of different drugs to optimize pain treatment (such as local anesthetics for continuous peripheral nerve blocks, opioids, nonsteroidal anti-inflammatory drugs). The roles played by the different specialists must be coordinated to optimize the rehabilitation of the patient after surgery.

Accordingly, both ward nurses and those involved in the postoperative care of patients need to be trained to ensure that all care givers know how to run a pump, order and change bags of local anesthetic mixtures, and who to call in case of problems. Prior to the use of a continuous block technique, these different steps must be carefully followed:

- Adequate medical examination of the patient, to assess the neurological condition, especially in relation to preexisting deficits in sensory and motor function in the territory involved by the block. A bilateral examination is always recommended.

The catheter is secured to the skin with Stery-strips.

▼ **Figure 6.1**

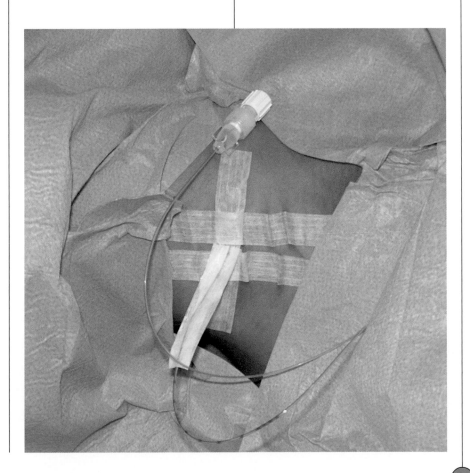

- Discuss with the patient the risk of neurological complications associated with this technique and verify with the patient that he or she has a complete understanding of the possible neurological complications also associated with surgery and positioning during the procedure.
- Always use appropriate monitoring and venous access during the procedure.
- Provide the same sedation as for a single block (minimum to moderate). The placement of a perineural catheter is contraindicated in anesthetized patients, except for infants and children and in patients receiving a continuous lumbar plexus catheter for postoperative pain control after open reduction internal fixation for an acetabular fracture.
- Prepare the drugs required for the postoperative infusion before the patient leaves the operating room, to ensure that the infusion is initiated as soon as possible upon arrival in the post anesthesia care unit.
- If the anesthetic block is also required for the surgery, an initial injection through the introducing needle is recommended before placement of the catheter.
- Secure the catheter to the skin effectively. For some approaches, such as the interscalene or the axillary approach, associated with frequent displacement of the

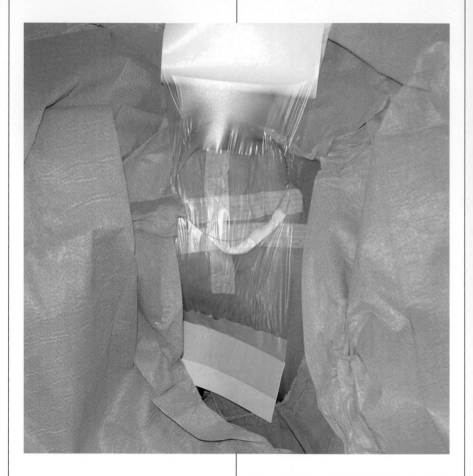

▲ **Figure 6.2**

The catheter insertion site is covered with a transparent Tegaderm®.

catheter, a 2–3 cm tunnelization can be used to minimize the risk of dislocation. New devices are now available to facilitate how catheters are secured to the skin. In our experience we obtain very good results by securing the catheter in place with 12 mm × 100 mm Stery-strips (3M Health

Care, St Paul, MN, USA; *Figure 6.1*). The catheter is then covered with a transparent Tegaderm (3M Health Care, St Paul, MN, USA; *Figure 6.2*). A transparent dressing is preferable because it allows a direct and easy evaluation of the insertion site during the postoperative period.

BRACHIAL PLEXUS

F. Alemanno, L. Bertini, A. Casati, P. Di Benedetto

■ Anatomy

The brachial plexus derives from the anterior primary rami of C5, C6, C7, C8, and T1, with contributions from C4 and T2 nerves. After leaving their intervertebral foramina, these nerves run laterally and caudally, lying between the anterior and middle scalene muscles and descending toward the first rib. Just above the first rib the roots of C5 and C6 fuse to form the superior trunk, the roots of C8 and T1 fuse to form the inferior trunk, and the root of C7 continues between these two trunks as the middle trunk of the brachial plexus *(Figure 7.1)*. The prevertebral fascia covers both scalene muscles, enclosing the brachial plexus in a fascial sheath.

At the lateral edge of the first rib, each trunk forms anterior and posterior divisions that run toward the axilla. Interestingly, the fibers contained in the anterior divisions innervate the anterior surface of the upper extremity and shoulder, while those contained in the posterior divisions innervate the posterior surface of the limb. In the axilla

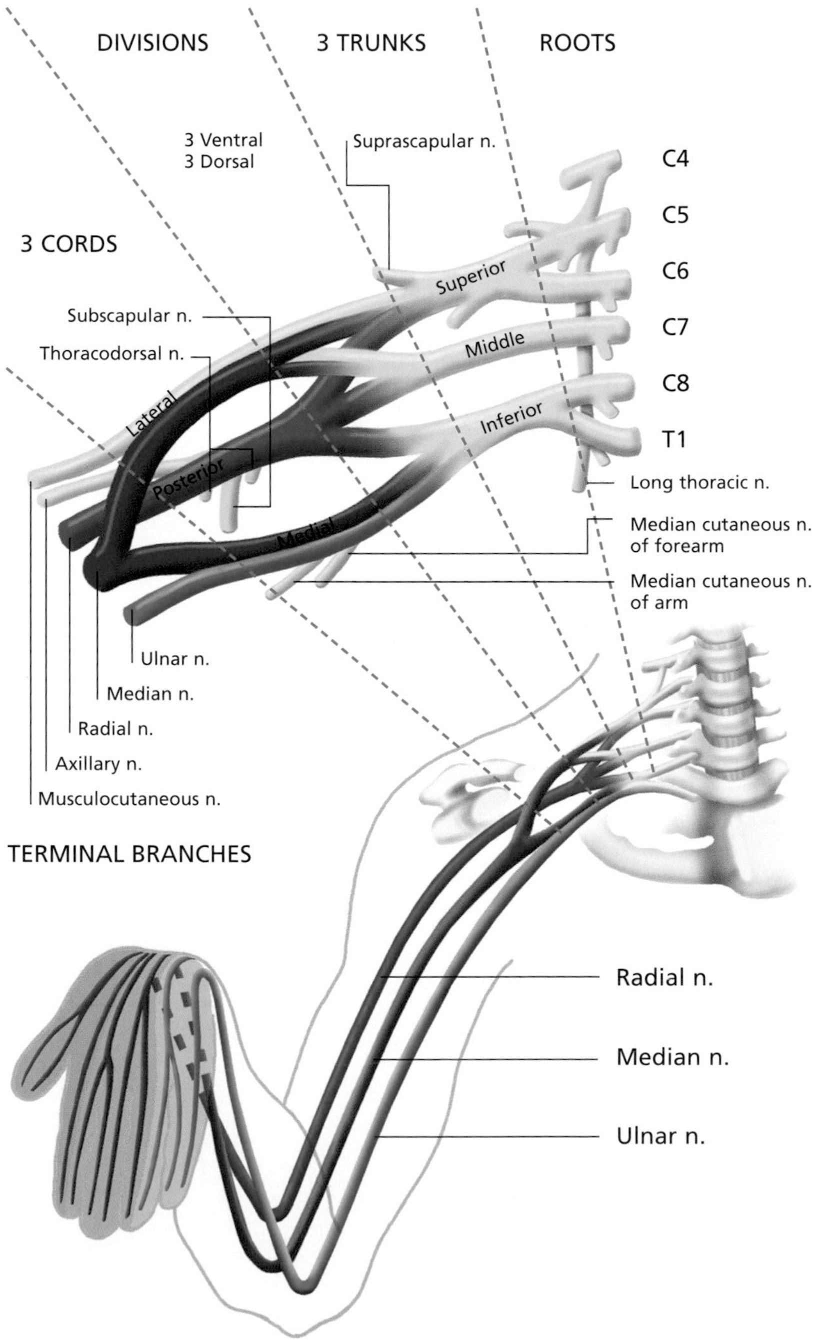

DIVISIONS   3 TRUNKS   ROOTS

3 Ventral
3 Dorsal

Suprascapular n.

C4

C5

3 CORDS

Superior

C6

Subscapular n.

Middle

C7

Thoracodorsal n.

C8

Lateral

Inferior

T1

Posterior

Long thoracic n.

Medial

Median cutaneous n. of forearm

Median cutaneous n. of arm

Ulnar n.

Median n.

Radial n.

Axillary n.

Musculocutaneous n.

TERMINAL BRANCHES

Radial n.

Median n.

Ulnar n.

Brachial plexus anatomy.

Figure 7.1 ▶

these divisions form lateral, posterior, and medial cords according to their position with respect to the axillary artery.

Finally, at the lateral border of the pectoralis minor, the three cords divide into the terminal peripheral nerves of the upper extremity:

- the lateral cord provides the lateral portion of the median nerve and the musculocutaneous nerve;
- the medial cord provides the medial portion of the median nerve, the ulnar nerve, the medial antebrachial nerve, and the medial brachial cutaneous nerve; and

- the posterior cord divides into the axillary and radial nerves.

The rationale for blocking the brachial plexus is based on the presence of a sheath in which the brachial plexus nerves are contained, from the intervertebral foramina to the distal axilla. Consequently, the brachial plexus can be blocked at different levels from the neck to the axilla. Beyond the axilla the nerves are separated and have to be blocked individually (mid-humeral approach, elbow and wrist blocks).

Injecting a large volume of local anesthetic solution could theoretically spread throughout the sheath and produce a block of the brachial plexus, irrespective of the site of injection. However, it is well established that each approach results in a preferential distribution, anesthesia, and postoperative analgesia.

Thus, the choice of approach must be based on the type and level at which the surgery is performed. The most frequently used approaches for a continuous block of the upper limb are interscalene, infraclavicular, and axillary.

Continuous interscalene block

Landmarks

The patient is placed in a supine position with the head slightly turned away from the operated side. The interscalene groove, formed by the anterior and middle scalene muscles, is palpated at the level of the cricoid cartilage (C6). This can be facilitated by palpating the poste-

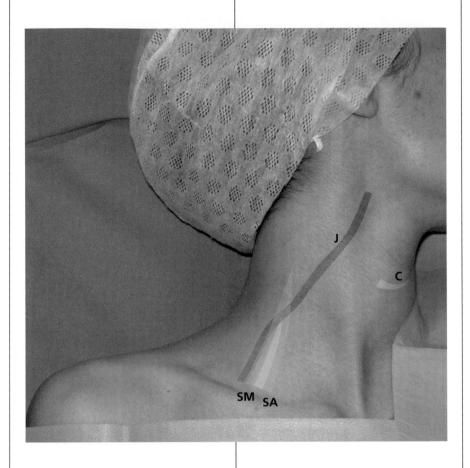

Landmarks for interscalene brachial plexus block.

   SA: anterior scalene muscle;

   SM: medium scalene muscle;

   J: external jugular vein;

   C: cricoid cartilage.

Figure 7.2 ▶

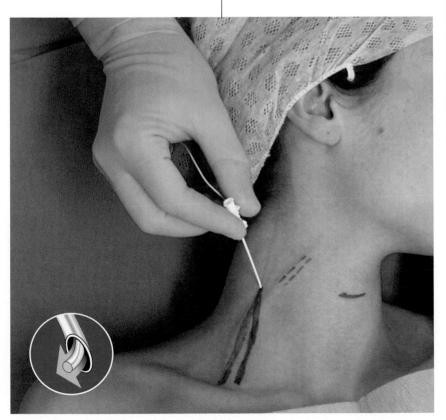

rior border of the sternocleidomastoid muscle and rolling the finger laterally and posteriorly to feel the scalene muscle. If the groove is not palpated the patient may be asked to take a slow and deep breath to facilitate the location of the scalene muscle.

The apex of the triangle formed by the two scalene muscles is drawn on the skin. The needle insertion site is at the level of the cricoid cartilage *(Figure 7.2)*.

Technique for the placement of an interscalene catheter for continuous brachial plexus block. The bevel of the Tuohy needle is directed toward the axilla. (The arrow in the inset circle indicates the direction of the catheter.)

◀ **Figure 7.3**

Technique

After appropriate skin disinfection and local infiltration with 2 ml of lidocaine 1%, a 3.75–5 cm insulated Tuohy needle, connected to a nerve stimulator (stimulating current intensity 1–1.5 mA, frequency 2 Hz), is inserted in a caudal and slightly posterior direction.

The needle is introduced at a 45° angle until either a contraction of the deltoid muscle or a contraction of the biceps muscle with elbow flexion is elicited.

Once the required muscular twitch is observed, the stimulating intensity is progressively reduced, while the needle position is adjusted to maintain an adequate motor response with a current ≤0.5 mA. Then, after negative aspiration for blood, 30–40 ml of local anesthetic solution (ropivacaine 0.5–0.75%, or a 1/1 mixture of mepivacaine 1.5% and ropivacaine 0.75%) is injected slowly in 5 ml increments with multiple aspirations for blood to exclude intravascular injection. Afterward, a 20-gauge epidural catheter is introduced through the Tuohy needle, 3–4 cm from the tip *(Figure 7.3)*.

The needle is removed and the catheter secured to the skin. To minimize the risk of displacement of the catheter, since the interscalene groove is very superficial, the catheter is tunneled for 2–3 cm using an 18-gauge intravenous cannula.

Postoperatively, the catheter is infused with ropivacaine 0.2% at an infusion rate of 8–12 ml/h. With a patient-controlled analgesia technique, a basal infusion rate of 5 ml/h with a 2.5 ml bolus and a 30 minute lockout time is used.

Indications

A continuous interscalene brachial plexus block is indicated for rotator cuff and open shoulder surgery, for both anesthesia and postoperative analgesia, as well as for procedures that involve the proximal part of the upper limb.

The diffusion of local anesthetic solution toward the inferior part of the cervical plexus (C4) improves the quality of pain control for shoulder procedures.

This approach can provide analgesia to the forearm also, but it must be emphasized that the diffusion of local anesthetic to the inferior trunk is usually incomplete, which prevents the distribution of good analgesia and/or anesthesia to the ulnar nerve *(Figure 7.4)*.

A continuous interscalene block produces a very good sympathetic block, and so can be used for algodystrophy and chronic pain syndromes.

Tips

- If a contraction of the trapezius muscle is elicited the needle is withdrawn to the skin and redirected anteriorly.
- If a contraction of the ipsilateral hemidiaphragm is elicited, the stimulating needle is withdrawn to the skin and redirected posteriorly.
- Single interscalene block always produces a paresis of the ipsilateral hemidiaphragm. The block of the ipsilateral hemidiaphragm is nearly constant during continuous interscalene block (in nearly 75% of cases) and is maintained throughout the infusion period in nearly 50% of patients. In healthy patients, block of the ipsilateral hemidiaphragm does not result in any significant change in the patient's oxygenation; however, a continuous block of the diaphragm should be avoided in patients with severe respiratory disease. The degree of motor block is affected by the concentration of the anesthetic solution. Bupivacaine 0.125% affects pulmonary function less than bupivacaine 0.25%. Ropivacaine 0.2% has markedly less effect on the motor function as compared with equipotent doses of bupivacaine.
- Diffusion of the anesthetic solution to the cervical sympathetic nervous system frequently produces a Claude–Bernard–Horner syndrome.
- Some authors have reported an unintended cannulation of the vertebral artery, with associated systemic toxicity. For this reason it is always important to verify negative blood aspiration before starting the infusion.

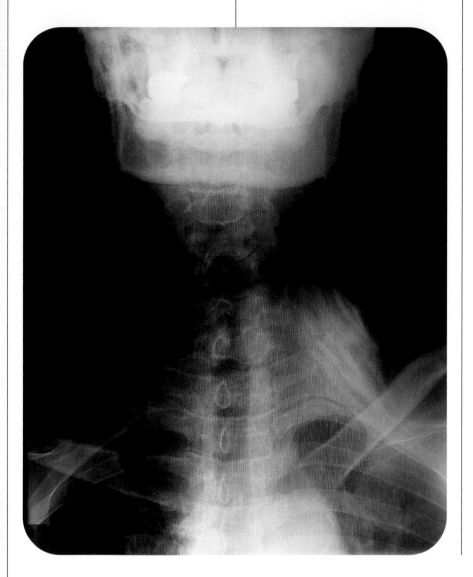

Figure 7.4

Radiographic visualization of an appropriate placement of an interscalene catheter after surgery.

Continuous supraclavicular block according to Alemanno

Landmarks

The approach to the brachial plexus according to Alemanno's technique produces a good block of the shoulder and upper limb.

The main landmarks are given by the pulse of the subclavian artery posteriorly to the midpoint of the clavicle (*Figure 7.5*). Another useful landmark is the spinous process of C7.

Technique

After appropriate skin disinfection and local infiltration with 2 ml of lidocaine 1%, a 3.75–5 cm insulated Tuohy needle is inserted nearly 0.5 cm laterally to the pulse of the subclavian artery and then advanced in a posteromedial direction toward the spinous process of C7. Skin puncture with an 18-gauge needle after the local infiltration needle has been removed can facilitate introduction of the Tuohy needle (*Figure 7.6*).

The nerve stimulator is set at 1 mA, and the Tuohy needle is advanced along the C7 plane until an appropriate muscular twitch (usually contraction of the deltoid or biceps muscle) is elicited. Once this is observed, the stimulating current is progressively reduced to 0.3–0.4 mA, adjusting the needle position to maintain the correct motor response. Then, after negative aspiration for blood, 30–40 ml of anesthetic solution is injected slowly with a repeated aspiration for blood test every 5 ml. After this a 20-gauge catheter is introduced through the needle 3–4 cm from the tip.

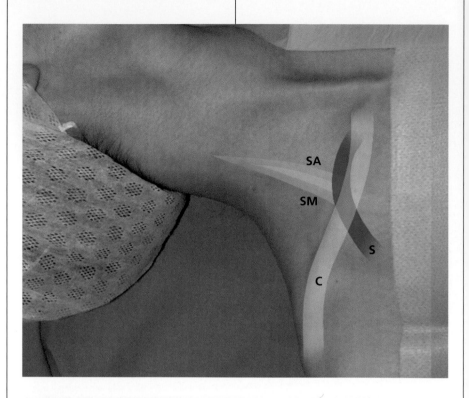

▲ **Figure 7.5**

Landmarks for the Alemanno supraclavicular block.
SA: anterior scalene muscle;
SM: medium scalene muscle;
C: clavicle;
S: subclavian artery.

The catheter is secured to the skin after removing the needle. With this approach a 2–3 cm tunnel can also help to optimize the catheter fixation.

Postoperatively, the catheter is usually infused with ropivacaine 0.2% (6–10 ml/h). If a patient-controlled analgesia technique is used the pump is set at 5–6 ml/h, with a bolus of 2.5 ml and a 30 minute lockout period (*Figure 7.7*).

Indications

This approach is indicated for surgical procedures that involve the shoulder and the arm down to the elbow.

Tips

- The direction of needle insertion described with this approach minimizes the risk of pneumothorax compared with the classic supraclavicular approach.
- This part of the body is minimally exposed to movement after surgery, which reduces the risk of catheter displacement.

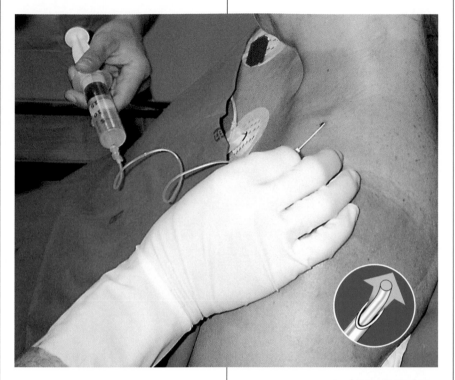

◄ Figure 7.6
Brachial plexus block with the Alemanno supraclavicular approach. (The arrow in the inset circle indicates the direction of the catheter.)

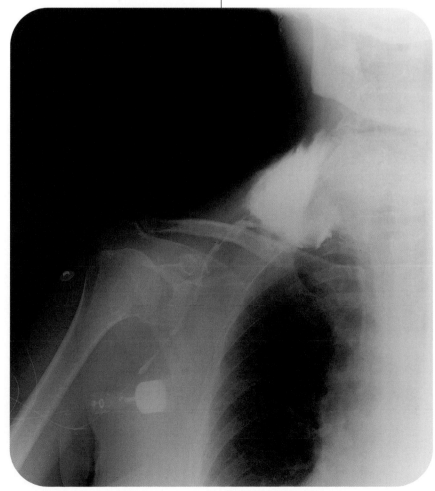

Radiographic visualization of the distribution of 15 ml of dye solution injected through a supraclavicular catheter.

Figure 7.7 ▶

Continuous infraclavicular block

Landmarks

The infraclavicular approach to the brachial plexus block enables the anesthetic solution to be placed around the trunk *(Figures 7.1 and 7.8)*. Compared to the supraclavicular approaches, the infraclavicular approach is associated with a lower risk of pleural puncture. The landmarks for infraclavicular approaches to the brachial plexus are Chassaignac's tubercle, the midpoint of the clavicle, the pulse of the axillary artery and/or the groove between the deltoid and pectoralis major muscles.

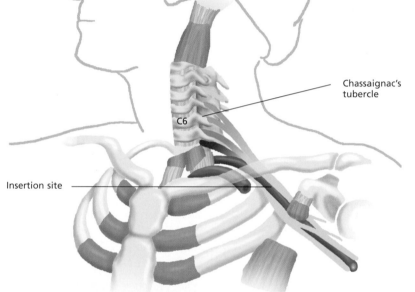

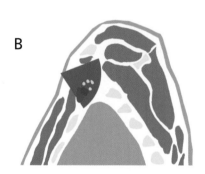

Chassaignac's tubercle

C6

Insertion site

▲ **Figure 7.8**

Anatomy of the brachial plexus at the infraclavicular level (A), and horizontal section (B).

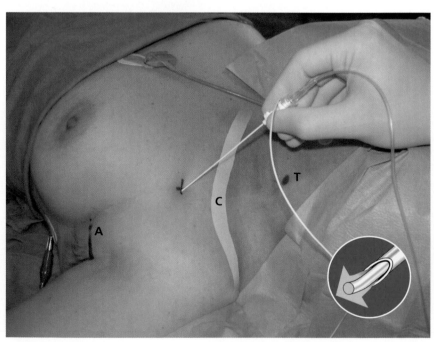

Landmarks for infraclavicular brachial plexus block (classic Raj's approach).
- *T: Chassaignac's tubercle;*
- *A: axillary artery.*
- *C: clavicle.*
(The arrow in the inset circle indicates the direction of the catheter.)

Figure 7.9 ▶

Technique

Two different approaches can be used for catheter placement, the classic Raj's approach or the vertical approach. For Raj's approach, the patient is placed in a supine position with the arm to be blocked abducted 90° at the shoulder. If this is not possible, the arm can be mantained in a neutral position and the groove between the deltoid and pectoralis muscles can be used instead of the pulse of the axillary artery. For the vertical approach, the arm remains in a neutral position along the body.

In both approaches the head is turned slightly away from the operated side.

Classic Raj's approach. The midpoint of the clavicle, and the axillary artery are marked on the skin.

Needle insertion site is 2.5 cm below the midclavicle point *(Figures 7.8 and 7.9)*.

With the physician at the head of the patient and after local infiltra-

tion with 2–3 ml of lidocaine 1%, a 10–15 cm insulated Tuohy needle is inserted at 45°. The nerve stimulator is set to deliver a current of intensity 1–1.5 mA and frequency 2 Hz while the needle is advanced toward the pulse of the axillary artery until the required motor response is elicited at the level of the wrist or fingers (flexion, extension, adduction). The intensity of the stimulating current is progressively reduced to ≤0.5 mA, adjusting the needle position to maintain the proper motor response. Then 30–40 ml of local anesthetic solution (ropivacaine 0.5–0.75%, or a 1/1 mixture of mepivacaine 1.5% and ropivacaine 0.75%) is injected slowly after negative aspiration for blood; aspiration must be repeated at every 5 ml increment. Afterward, a 20-gauge epidural catheter is introduced through the Tuohy needle 3–4 cm from the tip toward the apex of the axilla. The needle is then removed and the catheter secured to the skin.

Vertical approach. The brachial plexus can also be reached below the clavicle with a vertical approach *(Figure 7.8)*. The landmark is the inferior border of the midpoint of the clavicle. A 5 cm insulated Tuohy needle is inserted 1 cm below this point perpendicular to the skin, and then advanced for no more than 3–4 cm, with the bevel turned toward the apex of the axilla *(Figure 7.10)*, until an appropriate muscular twitch is elicited at the level of the wrist or fingers (flexion, extension, adduction).

Postoperatively, irrespective of the approach used, the catheter is usually infused with ropivacaine 0.2% (6–10 ml/h). If a patient-controlled analgesia technique is used the pump is set at 5–6 ml/h, with a bolus of 2.5 ml and a 30 minute lockout period.

Indications

The infraclavicular block can be used for anesthesia and postoperative analgesia for surgery involving the humerus, elbow, forearm, wrist, and hand. It is very useful for patients who require prolonged postoperative analgesia, such as trauma patients, those undergoing reimplantation of the extremity, or those with vascular diseases or chronic pain syndromes.

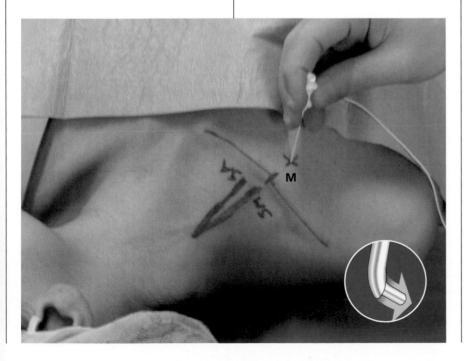

Landmarks for the infraclavicular brachial plexus block with a vertical approach.
  SA: anterior scalene muscle;
  SM: medium scalene muscle;
  M: midpoint of the clavicle.
(The arrow in the inset circle indicates the direction of the catheter.)

◄ **Figure 7.10**

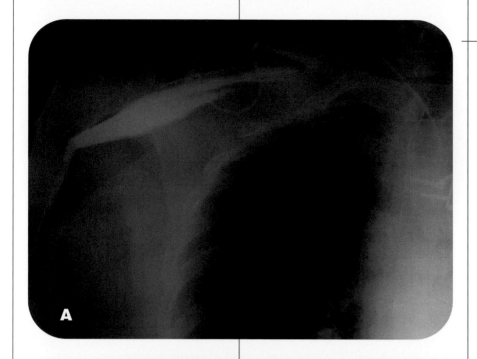

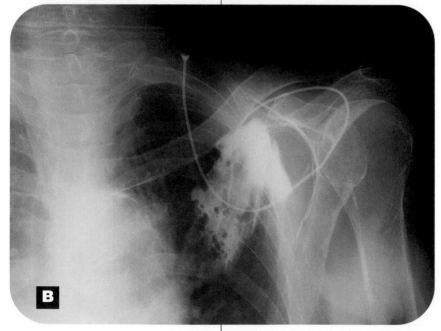

Tips

- The musculocutaneous nerve leaves the sheath of the brachial plexus early. For this reason the catheter must be placed after eliciting a motor response, at the level of the wrist or fingers *(Figure 7.11)*.

- The infraclavicular approach does not block the phrenic nerve, and so avoids the negative effects on pulmonary function produced by the interscalene approach. Thus it can also be used in patients with lung disease.

- Another advantage of this approach is that it can be performed even if the patient cannot abduct the arm. In such cases a vertical approach can be used.

- These approaches are also indicated for procedures requiring infusions longer than 48–72 hours. These catheters can be easily maintained for up to 2–3 weeks.

- A disadvantage is the increased risk of axillary artery puncture.

▲ **Figure 7.11**

A) Radiographic visualization of an appropriately placed infraclavicular catheter.

B) Placement of an infraclavicular catheter outside the brachial plexus sheath: in this case the catheter was placed after eliciting a stimulation of the musculocutaneous nerve.

Continuous axillary block

The axillary approach for continuous brachial plexus block has been described and used since the early 1970s. It can also be used easily for pediatric patients.

Landmarks

The axilla is a pyramid-shaped space. The base is the concave armpit, the anterior wall is formed by the pectoral muscles, the posterior wall comprises the scapula and subscapular muscles, the lateral wall is formed by the medial part of the humerus, and the medial wall is formed by ribs 1–4. The apex is formed by the border of the first rib, the superior border of the scapula and the posterior part of the clavicle. At the level of the axilla, the trunks of the brachial plexus are already divided into their posterior and anterior divisions, which originate the lateral, medial, and posterior cords *(Figure 7.1)*.

The axillary artery is surrounded by nerves within the sheath, while at the level of the distal axilla the artery is surrounded by the terminal branches of the plexus (the radial, ulnar, and median nerves).

The musculocutaneous nerve leaves the axilla proximally and enters the coracobrachial muscle.

The radial nerve is usually found posterior to the axillary artery, the ulnar nerve lies on the inferior or posterior border of the axillary artery, and the median nerve lies on the superior surface of the axillary artery.

The landmarks are represented by the axillary artery, the inferior border of the major pectoralis muscle, and the long head of the biceps muscle *(Figure 7.12)*.

Technique

The patient is placed in the supine position, with the arm to be blocked abducted at about 90º, and the forearm flexed on the arm at 90º.

After appropriate skin disinfection and local infiltration with 2–3 ml of lidocaine 1%, a 5 cm insulated Tuohy needle is inserted at 45º.

The nerve stimulator is set to deliver a current of intensity 1–1.5 mA and frequency 2 Hz while the needle is advanced toward the pulse of the axillary artery until the required motor response is elicited at the level of the wrist or fingers (flexion, extension, adduction). The intensity of the stimulating current is progressively reduced to ≤0.5 mA,

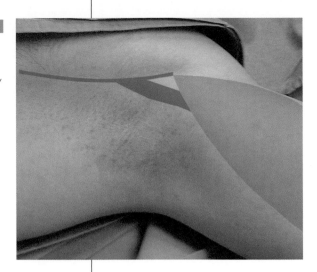

Figure 7.12 ▶

Landmarks for axillary catheter placement.

Red: pulse of the axillary artery;

Blue: border of the pectoralis muscle;

Pink: long head of the biceps muscle.

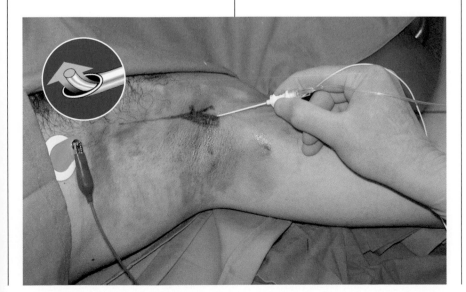

Continuous axillary plexus block.
(The arrow in the inset circle indicates the direction of the catheter.)

◀ **Figure 7.13**

Figure 7.14

Radiographic visualization of the distribution of 15–20 ml of dye solution (5 ml iopamidol diluted in 15 ml normal saline) injected through an axillary catheter.

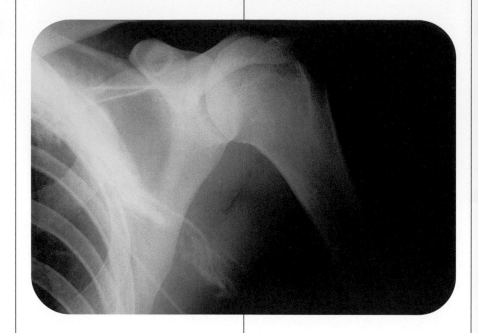

adjusting the needle position to maintain the motor response.

After negative aspiration for blood, 30–40 ml of local anesthetic solution (ropivacaine 0.5–0.75%, or a 1/1 mixture of mepivacaine 1.5% and ropivacaine 0.75%) is injected slowly with repeated aspirations for blood every 5 ml *(Figures 7.13 and 7.14)*.

A 20-gauge epidural catheter is introduced through the Tuohy needle 3–4 cm toward the apex of the axilla. The needle is removed and the catheter secured to the skin. Postoperatively, the catheter is usually infused with ropivacaine 0.2% (6–10 ml/h). If a patient-controlled analgesia technique is used, the pump is set at 5–6 ml/h, with a bolus of 2.5 ml and a 30 minute lockout period.

Indications

The axillary brachial plexus block is the most widely used continuous approach, and is considered by many to be the easiest and safest. It can be used for patients undergoing wrist, forearm, and hand surgery.

Other indications are vascular diseases and chronic pain syndromes *(Figure 7.14)*.

Tips

• To maximize the success rate, it is important to seek the specific motor response from the nerve involved by the surgery.

• At the level of the axilla, the brachial plexus is very superficial. Consequently, the catheter is tunneled to minimize the incidence of catheter displacement.

• The most frequent problem with the axillary block is an incomplete block of the musculocutaneous nerve. If the block is also used to provide anesthesia, it might be useful to carry out a separate block of the musculocutaneous nerve with an injection of 5 ml of anesthetic solution after eliciting an appropriate musculocutaneous-mediated muscular response with a nerve stimulator (flexion of the forearm).

LUMBAR PLEXUS AND FEMORAL NERVE

A. Casati, J.E. Chelly, G. Fanelli

■ Anatomy

The ventral rami of the first three lumbar nerves and part of the fourth form the lumbar plexus. Frequently, there is also a contribution from part of the 12th thoracic nerve. The obturator, femoral, and lateral femoral cutaneous nerves originate from the intervertebral foramina and run in the psoas muscle *(Figure 8.1)*. The femoral nerve divides into four main branches at or below the inguinal ligament:

- the vastus lateralis nerves follow a branch of the lateral femoral artery and supplies the vastus lateralis muscle;
- the vastus intermedius nerve runs along the surface of the vastus intermedius and innervates it;
- the vastus medialis nerve originates close to the saphenous nerve, enters the superior part of the quadriceps muscle, and supplies innervation to the vastus medialis muscle; and
- the saphenous nerve provides sensory innervation for the medial aspect of the leg and ankle.

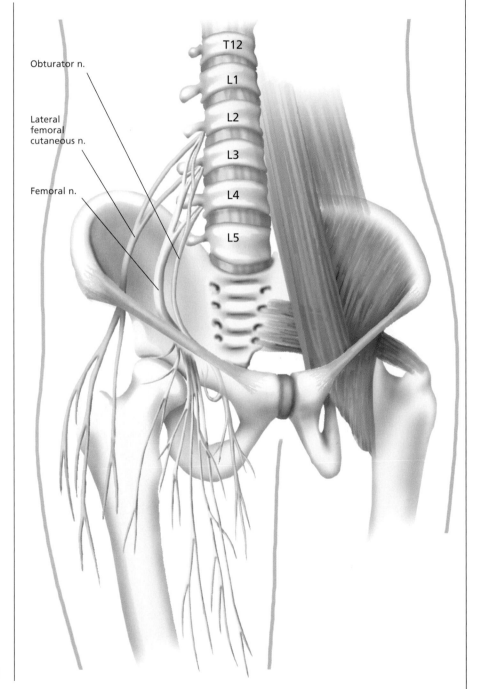

Obturator n.

Lateral femoral cutaneous n.

Femoral n.

T12
L1
L2
L3
L4
L5

Lumbar plexus anatomy.

Figure 8.1 ▶

For a continuous lumbar plexus block, a perineural catheter can be placed posteriorly at the level of the lumbar plexus or anteriorly at the level of the femoral nerve sheath.

A continuous lumbar plexus block is indicated for anesthesia and acute postoperative pain management in hip surgery, acetabular fractures, and operations that involve the proximal part of the femur and the knee.

A continuous femoral block is mainly indicated for surgical proce- dures that involve the knee, such as knee arthroplasty, anterior cruciate ligament repair, and open reduc- tion and fixation of a patella frac- ture. It has also been advocated for hip arthroplasty.

Continuous lumbar plexus block

Landmarks

A catheter can be placed at the level of the lumbar plexus using either a loss-of-resistance technique or a nerve stimulator. Our technique combines both approaches. The patient is placed in the lateral decubitus position with the operated side up and the hips and knees slightly flexed to facilitate patient comfort.

The spinous processes of L2–L5 are identified and marked, and a vertical line is drawn at the level of the superior border of the posterior iliac crests (bisiliac line).

The site of needle introduction is located and marked, 5 cm lateral to the spinous process on the vertical line (*Figure 8.2*).

Technique

After appropriate local infiltration using a 25-gauge 3.75 cm needle and 2 ml lidocaine 1%, a 10 cm insulated Tuohy needle, connected to a 10 ml loss-of-resistance syringe and to a nerve stimulator (stimulating current intensity 1–1.5 mA, frequency 2 Hz), is introduced perpendicular to the skin. The tip of the Tuohy needle is oriented cephalad (*Figure 8.3*).

First, contractions of the iliocostalis lumborum muscle and of the paravertebral muscles are usually observed; within 6–8 cm, contractions of the paravertebral muscles disappear and loss of resistance in the syringe usually occurs, which indicates that the needle has reached the psoas compartment. At this point, or slightly deeper, contraction of the

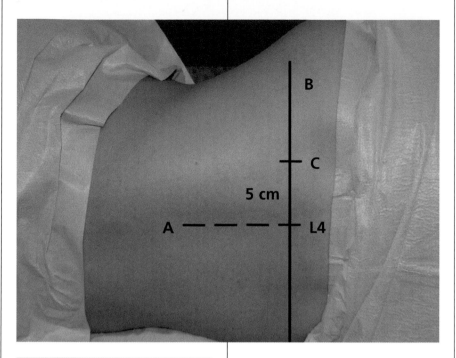

▲ **Figure 8.2**

Landmarks for lumbar plexus block.
   A: interspinous line;
   B: bisiliac line;
   I: insertion site, 5 cm lateral to the interspinous line on the bisiliac line.

Posterior approach to the lumbar plexus. The stimulating needle, connected to a nerve stimulator, is inserted perpendicular to the skin.

Combination with a loss of resistance technique may help. (The arrow in the inset circle indicates the direction of the catheter.)

▼ **Figure 8.3**

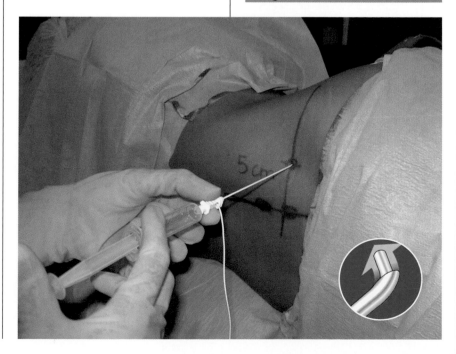

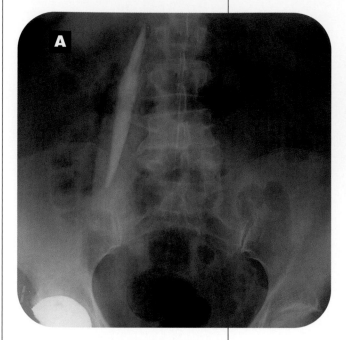

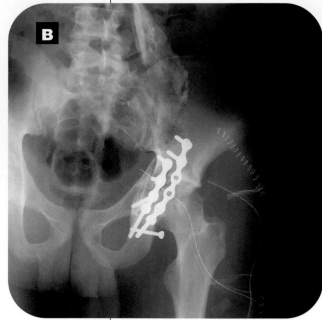

▲ **Figure 8.4**

Radiographic visualization of the correct placement of a continuous lumbar plexus block after hip surgery (A) or open reduction and internal fixation of acetabular fracture (B).

quadriceps muscle is elicited; the position of the needle is adjusted to mantain the same motor response with a current of ≤0.5 mA.

After negative aspiration for blood, 20–30 ml of a local anesthetic solution (ropivacaine 0.5–0.75%, or a 1/1 mixture of mepivacaine 1.5% and ropivacaine 0.75%) is slowly injected in 5 ml increments with multiple aspirations to exclude intravascular injection. Afterwards, a 20-gauge epidural catheter is introduced through the Tuohy needle 3–4 cm into the psoas compartment. If the block is used in combination with a sciatic nerve block, to minimize the risk of overdosing, consideration should be given to the total volume of local anesthetic (no more than 40–50 ml total volume). The catheter is secured to the skin.

A continuous infusion of ropivacaine 0.2% is used postoperatively at an infusion rate of 8–12 ml/h. If a patient-controlled analgesia technique is used, the infusion rate is set at 5–8 ml/h with a 2.5 ml bolus and a lockout period of 30 minutes.

Indications

Continuous lumbar plexus blocks are indicated, combined with a light general anesthetic, for surgery and postoperative analgesia in patients undergoing hip, thigh, and knee surgery.

For lower extremity surgery that involves the hip and for the thigh and/or knee, a combination of this block and a sciatic nerve block should be considered for anesthesia *(Figure 8.4)*.

Tips

- In most patients there is no need to introduce the stimulating Tuohy needle beyond 9 cm.

- The transverse process of L4 is often encountered, in which case the needle is walked cephalad off the transverse process for up to 2 cm, until a quadriceps contraction is elicited.

- The catheter should not be introduced more than 3–4 cm to minimize the risks of kinking and/or misplacement.

- There is a risk of epidural spread, especially if large volumes of local anesthetic are used.

  Consequently, it is important to inject the local anesthetic solution slowly and monitor vital signs carefully.

Figure 8.5 ▶

The lumbar plexus block may be a useful alternative when anatomical conditions prevent the placement of a central block as in this patient, in whom it was difficult to place an epidural catheter because of the marked scoliosis.

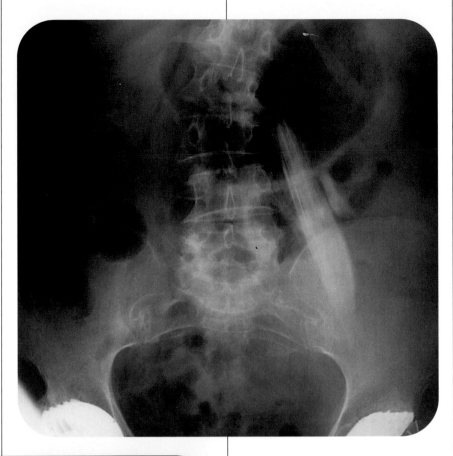

- Continuous lumbar plexus block is an effective and safe alternative to continuous epidural analgesia, especially when anticoagulants are given postoperatively or in patients in whom technical difficulties in locating the epidural space are expected *(Figures 8.5 and 8.6)*.

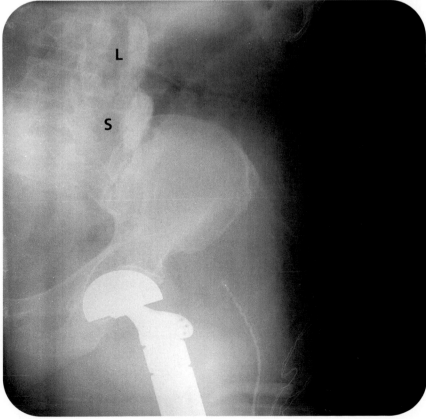

- The psoas compartment can also be located by using the loss-of-resistance technique alone; however, the use of a nerve stimulator increases the predictability of an appropriate catheter placement.

Diffusion of the dye solution not only at the lumbar plexus (L) but also at the sacral plexus (S) after the placement of a lumbar plexus catheter.

Continuous femoral nerve block

Landmarks

The patient is placed supine in a neutral position. Extra rotation of the leg to be blocked must be avoided. The needle insertion site is 1 cm lateral to the femoral artery at the level of the femoral crease *(Figure 8.7)*.

Technique

After appropriate local infiltration with 2 ml lidocaine 1%, a 5 cm insulated Tuohy needle, connected to a nerve stimulator (stimulating current intensity 1–1.5 mA, frequency 2 Hz), is introduced with

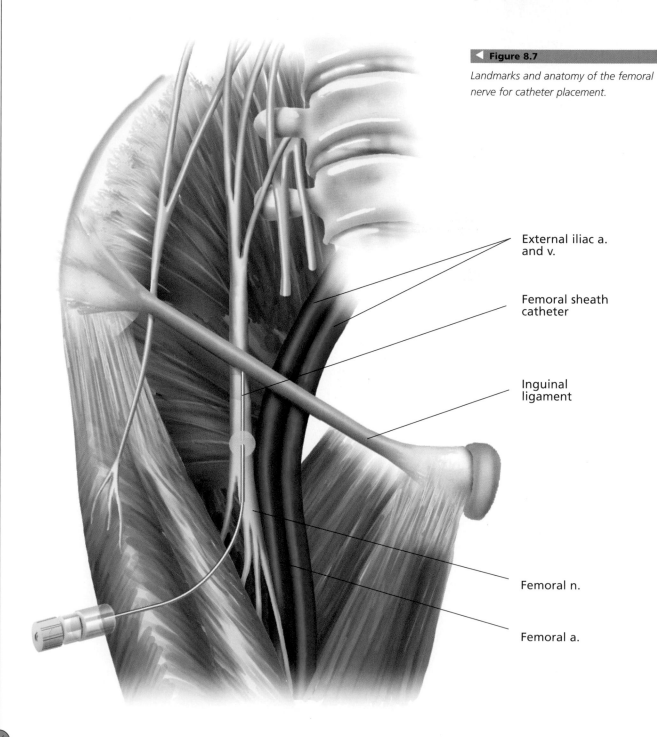

◀ **Figure 8.7**

Landmarks and anatomy of the femoral nerve for catheter placement.

External iliac a. and v.

Femoral sheath catheter

Inguinal ligament

Femoral n.

Femoral a.

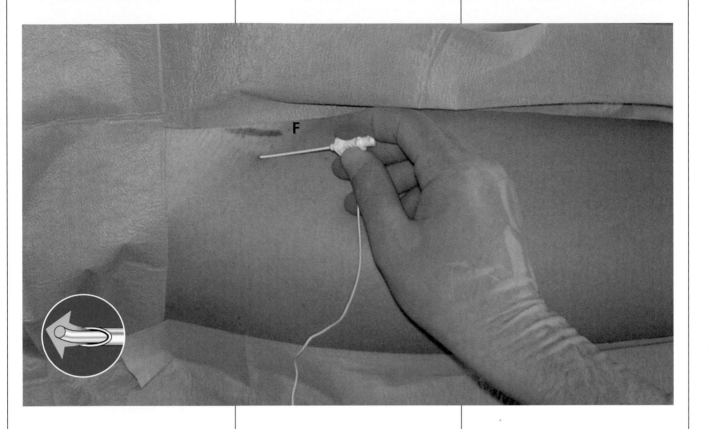

Landmarks for femoral nerve block.
  F: femoral artery.
(The arrow in the inset circle indicates the direction of the catheter.)

the tip oriented cephalad and at about 45° *(Figure 8.8)*.

The needle is advanced until movements of the patella are elicited. If contraction of the vastus medialis muscle is elicited, the needle is redirected slightly more laterally and deeper. The stimulating intensity is reduced progressively, while the needle position is adjusted to maintain the same motor response with a current of ≤0.5 mA.

Then, after negative aspiration for blood, 20–30 ml of local anesthetic solution (ropivacaine 0.5–0.75%, or a 1/1 mixture of mepivacaine 1.5% and ropivacaine 0.75%) is injected slowly in 5 ml increments with multiple aspiration tests. A 20-gauge epidural catheter is introduced through the Tuohy needle 3–4 cm from the tip. The needle is removed and the catheter secured to the skin. If the block is used in combination with a sciatic nerve block, to minimize the risk of overdosing consideration should be given to the total volume of anesthetic (no more than 40–50 ml total volume). A continuous infusion of ropivacaine 0.2% is used postoperatively at an infusion rate of 8–10 ml/h. If a patient-controlled analgesia technique is used the infusion rate is set at 5 ml/h with a 2.5 ml bolus and 30 minute lockout time.

Indications

Continuous femoral nerve block is indicated with a sciatic nerve block alone or combined with sedation to provide anesthesia for lower extremity surgery. Continuous femoral nerve block is also indicated for postoperative analgesia after thigh and knee surgery.

Figure 8.9 ▶

Radiographic visualization of 15 ml dye solution injected through a femoral catheter.

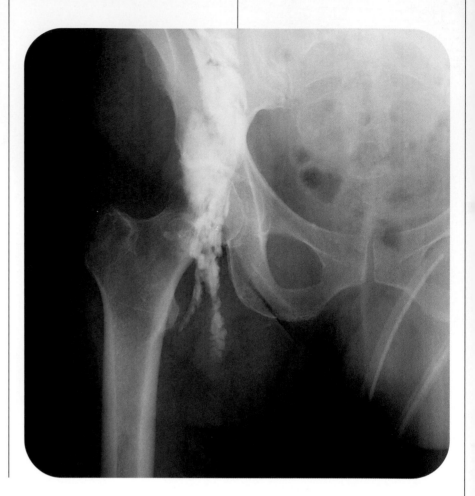

Tips

- The catheter can also be placed using an iliac fascia approach with a non-insulated Tuohy needle and a '2-pop' technique as the needle passes through the fascia lata and the fascia iliaca.
  Accordingly, the catheter is inserted below the fascia iliaca, after the second pop is felt.
- Introducing the catheter for 3–4 cm usually also produces a lateral femoral cutaneous and more frequently an obturator nerve block, which improves the quality of postoperative analgesia *(Figure 8.9)*.

SACRAL PLEXUS AND SCIATIC NERVE

A. Casati, J.E. Chelly, P. Di Benedetto, G. Fanelli

Anatomy

The ventral rami of the fourth lumbar to the fourth sacral spinal nerves form the sacral plexus. The nerves that enter the plexus converge to form a broad triangle, from which originate the sciatic nerve (L4–S3), the pudendal nerve (S2–S4), the superior gluteal nerve (L4–S1), and various other nerves for the pelvis and lower extremity. The sciatic nerve passes through the inferior part of the greater sciatic foramen, below the pirifom muscle and anterior to the gluteal region.

The sciatic nerve divides into the tibial nerve and common peroneal nerve at a variable point, but often these two nerves are distinct within the sheath of the sciatic nerve. The tibial nerve is usually located in the medial portion of the sciatic nerve, whereas the common peroneal nerve occupies the lateral portion *(Figure 9.1)*.

The sciatic nerve passes in the hollow between the ischial tuberosity and the greater trochanter and enters the thigh through the inferior border of the gluteus maximus, where the nerves to the hamstring muscles originate.

At the level of the popliteal fossa, the common peroneal and tibial nerves separate. The tibial nerve runs forward to the posterior part of the leg and foot; the common peroneal nerve exits the popliteal fossa, and runs around the head of the fibula to reach

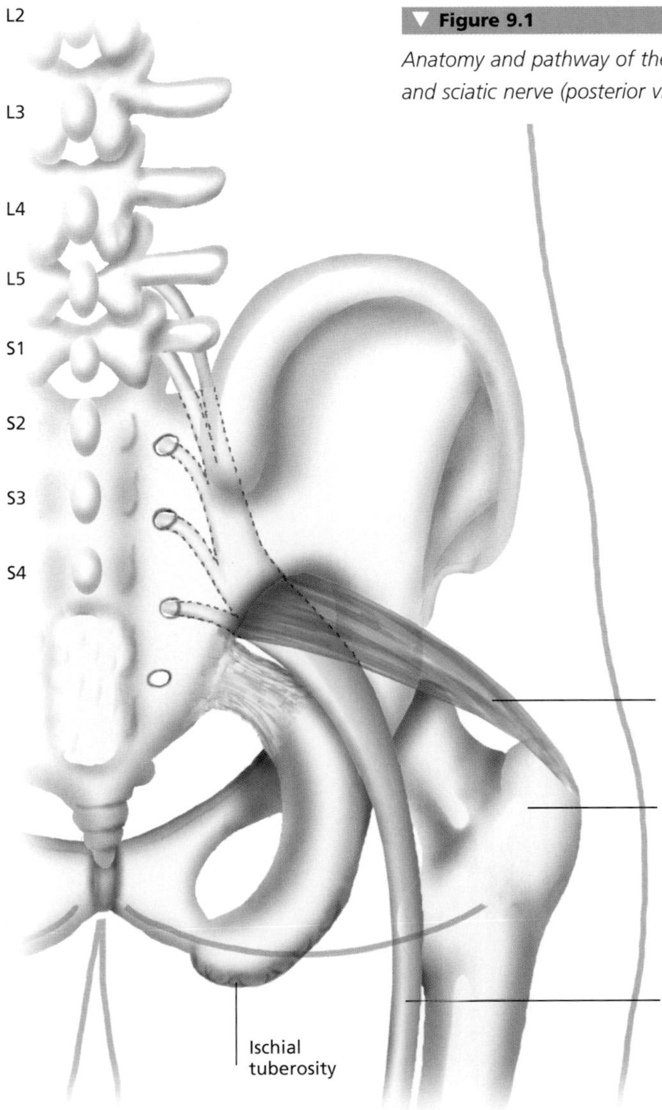

▼ **Figure 9.1**

Anatomy and pathway of the sacral plexus and sciatic nerve (posterior view).

L2
L3
L4
L5
S1
S2
S3
S4

Piriformis m.

Greater trochanter of femur

Sciatic n.

Ischial tuberosity

the lateral part of the leg and foot. A groove between the biceps femoris and semitendinous muscles can be identified, starting from 3 cm below the lower limit of the gluteus muscle, and continuing toward

the popliteal fossa. At the level of this groove lies the cutaneous projection of the sciatic nerve.

This identifies the 'sciatic line', along which the sciatic nerve can be reached at different levels.

■ Continuous parasacral block

Landmarks

The patient is placed in the lateral decubitus with the operated side up, and with the hips and knees slightly flexed to facilitate patient comfort. The posterior superior iliac spine and the ischial tuberosity are identified and a line drawn between these two points. The needle insertion site is 7 cm from the posterior superior iliac spine *(Figure 9.2)*.

Technique

After appropriate local infiltration with 2 ml lidocaine 1%, a 10 cm insulated Tuohy needle, connected to a nerve stimulator (stimulating current intensity 1–1.5 mA, frequency 2 Hz), is inserted perpendicular to the skin and advanced in a sagittal plane with the tip oriented laterally *(Figure 9.3)*.

If the sacrum is contacted, the needle is walked off the contour. Within 1–1.5 cm from this bone contact a proper sciatic stimulation is usually elicited [either the plantar flexion (tibial nerve) or dorsiflexion (common peroneal nerve)]. The needle position is then adjusted until an adequate muscular twitch is maintained with a stimulating current ≤0.5 mA. Then 20–30 ml of local anesthetic solution (ropivacaine 0.5–0.75%, or a 1/1 mixture of mepivacaine 1.5% and ropivacaine 0.75%) is injected slowly in 5 ml increments with multiple aspirations for blood.

At this point, a 20-gauge epidural catheter is introduced through the Tuohy needle 3–4 cm beyond its tip, after which the needle is removed and the catheter secured to the skin. If the block is used in

Landmarks for the parasacral sciatic block.
A: posterior superior iliac spine;
B: ischial tuberosity;
I: insertion site, 7 cm caudally to the iliac spine on the line connecting A to B.

▼ **Figure 9.2**

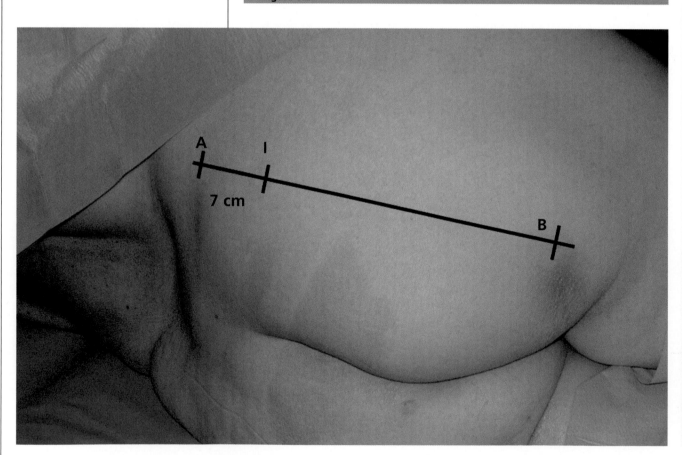

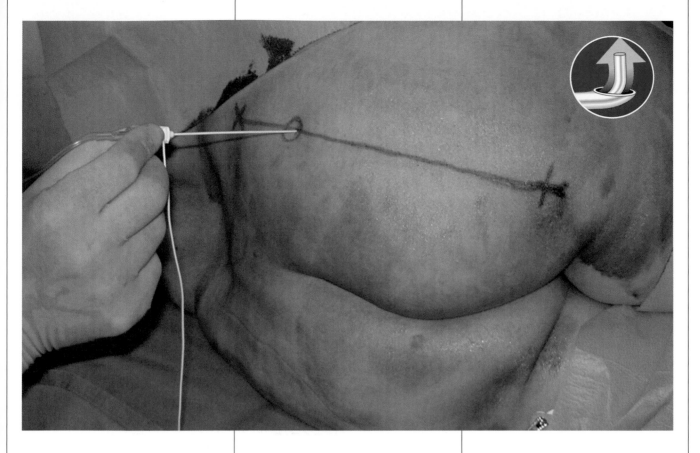

▲ **Figure 9.3**

Continuous parasacral block. (The arrow in the inset circle indicates the direction of the catheter.)

combination with a lumbar plexus block, to minimize the risk of overdosing consideration should be given to the total volume of anesthetic (no more than 40–50 ml total volume).

A continuous infusion of ropivacaine 0.2% is given postoperatively at an infusion rate of 5–8 ml/h. If a patient-controlled pump is used the infusion rate is set at 5 ml/h with a 2.5 ml bolus and 30 minute lockout period.

Indications

A continuous parasacral block is indicated, with a lumbar plexus block combined with sedation alone or with a light general anesthetic, for unilateral lower extremity surgery that involves the posterior aspect of the thigh. It is also indicated for acute postoperative pain control after surgery.

Tips

• Parasacral perineural infusion provides a true sacral continuous block, including a block of the posterior cutaneous femoral nerve of the thigh, which may be required especially for and after major surgery involving the posterior aspect of the thigh.

• The placement of a parasacral catheter reduces the risk of catheter misplacement or dislocation after surgery (compared with the classic Labat's approach), because of the absence of thick muscular layers at this level.

• To avoid injuries of pelvic organs, care must be taken to ensure the Tuohy needle is not introduced beyond 9 cm.

Continuous subgluteus sciatic nerve block according to Di Benedetto

Landmarks

Placement of a sciatic catheter using a posterior approach is usually painful because of the presence of a thick layer of muscles. In addition, the constant contraction of these muscles actually increases the probability of catheter displacement. At the level of the subgluteal region the sciatic nerve is included between the greater trochanter and the ischial tuberosity in the groove between the biceps femoris and semitendinous muscles, surrounded by a thinner layer of muscles.

According to Di Benedetto's approach (2001), the patient is placed in the lateral decubitus position, with the leg to be blocked up and rolled forward and the knee flexed at 90° (Sim's position). A line is drawn from the greater trochanter to the ischial tuberosity.

From the midpoint of this line a second line is drawn perpendicularly and extended caudally for 4 cm. This is the point of the needle entry *(Figure 9.4)*. At this level a skin depression, representing the groove between the biceps femoris and vastus lateralis muscles, is palpated.

Technique

After appropriate local skin infiltration with 2 ml lidocaine 1%, a 10 cm insulated Tuohy needle, connected to a nerve stimulator (stimulating current intensity 1–1.5 mA, frequency 2 Hz), is introduced with the tip oriented cephalad and at about 80º to the skin *(Figure 9.5)*.

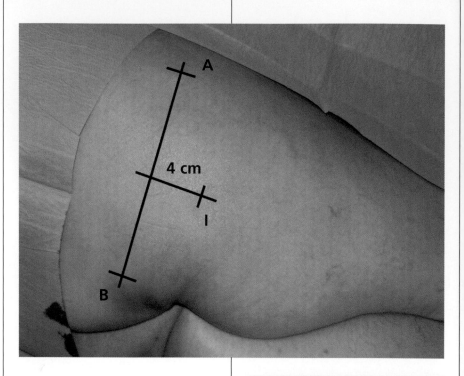

▲ Figure 9.4

Landmarks for the subgluteus sciatic block.
  A: greater trochanter;
  B: ischial tuberosity;
  I: insertion site, 4 cm caudally to the line connecting A to B, on a second line drawn perpendicularly from the midpoint of AB.

The Tuohy needle is advanced until either the plantar flexion (tibial nerve) or dorsiflexion (common peroneal nerve) is elicited. The needle position is adjusted until a proper motor response is maintained with a stimulating current ≤0.5 mA. After negative aspiration for blood, 20–30 ml of local anesthetic solution (ropivacaine 0.5–0.75%, or a 1/1 mixture of mepivacaine 1.5% and ropivacaine 0.75%) is injected slowly in 5 ml increments with multiple aspirations for blood. At this point, a 20-gauge epidural catheter is introduced through the Tuohy needle 3–4 cm beyond the tip, the needle is then removed, and the catheter is secured to the skin.

If the block is used in combination with a femoral nerve block, the volume of local anesthetic solution injected through the catheter must be reduced to minimize the risks of overdosing. A continuous infusion of ropivacaine 0.2% is used postoperatively at an infusion rate of 6–10 ml/h. If a patient-controlled pump is used the infusion rate is set at 5–7 ml/h with a 2.5 ml bolus and 30 minute lockout period *(Figure 9.6)*.

Indications

A continuous subgluteus sciatic nerve block is indicated with a femoral nerve block combined with sedation or light general anesthetic

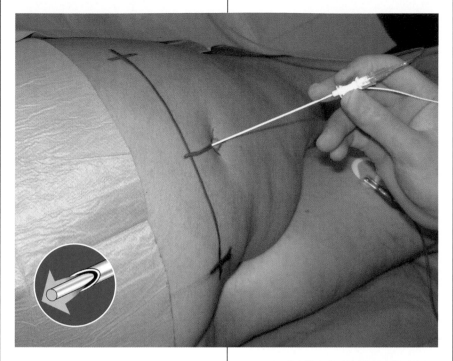

▲ **Figure 9.5**

Subgluteus approach. (The arrow in the inset circle indicates the direction of the catheter.)

for unilateral lower extremity surgery that involves the leg, ankle, and foot and requires more than 24 hours of postoperative pain control.

Tips

- The subgluteus approach reduces the risk of misplacement or dislocation after surgery, compared with the classic Labat's approach.
- To decrease the risk of displacement, the catheter can be tunneled laterally.
- Compared to popliteal approaches to the sciatic nerve, the risk of vascular puncture is lower with the subgluteus approach.

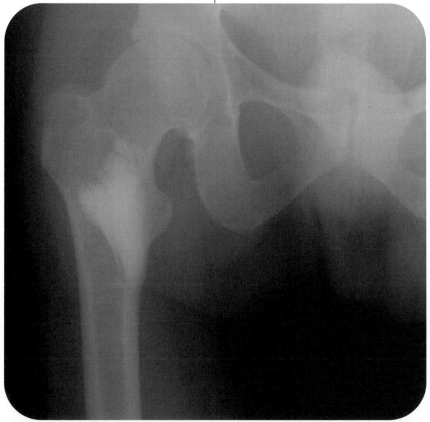

Radiographic visualization of an appropriate placement of a subgluteus sciatic catheter with dye solution.

▲ **Figure 9.6**

Continuous anterior sciatic nerve block according to Chelly

Landmarks

The sciatic nerve can also be reached anteriorly where it runs from the ischial tuberosity to the lesser trochanter.

With the patient in the supine position, a line is drawn from the lower border of the anterior superior iliac spine to the superolateral angle of the pubic tubercle. The midpoint of this line is used to draw a second perpendicular line. The site of insertion of the needle is 8 cm down this line *(Figure 9.7)*.

Technique

After appropriate local skin infiltration with 2 ml lidocaine 1% a 15 cm insulated Tuohy needle, connected to a nerve stimulator (stimulating current intensity 1–1.5 mA, frequency 2 Hz), is introduced with the tip oriented cephalad and perpendicular to the skin *(Figure 9.8)*. A contraction of the quadriceps muscle is often initially observed. To confirm that the needle is some distance from the femoral nerve, the intensity is reduced to 0.5 mA and the quadriceps contraction disappears. Then the needle is introduced another 1–2 cm, after which the intensity is set at 3–5 mA. The needle is advanced until a sciatic-mediated motor response occurs, via stimulation of either the common peroneal nerve (dorsiflexion eversion of the foot) or the tibial nerve (plantar flexion inversion of the foot and/or flexion of the toes).

The needle position is then adjusted until an adequate motor response is observed with a stimulating current ≤0.5 mA. After negative aspiration for blood, 20–30 ml of local anesthetic solution (ropivacaine 0.5–0.75%, or a 1/1 mixture of mepivacaine 1.5% and ropivacaine 0.75%) is injected slowly in 5 ml increments with multiple aspirations for blood. At this point, a 20-gauge epidural catheter is introduced through the Tuohy needle for 3–4 cm, with the needle tip oriented cranially, after which the needle is removed and the catheter secured to the skin.

If the block is used in combination with a femoral nerve block, the volume of local anesthetic solution injected through the catheter must be lowered to minimize the risks of overdosing. A continuous infusion of ropivacaine 0.2% is used postoperatively at an infusion rate of 6–10 ml/h. If a patient-controlled pump is used, the infusion rate is 5 ml/h with a 2.5 ml bolus and 30 minute lockout period.

Landmarks for the anterior sciatic block.
  A: lower border of the anterior superior iliac spine;
  B: superolateral angle of the pubic tubercle;
  I: insertion site, 8 cm caudally to the line connecting A to B on a line drawn perpendicularly from the midpoint of AB.

▼ **Figure 9.7**

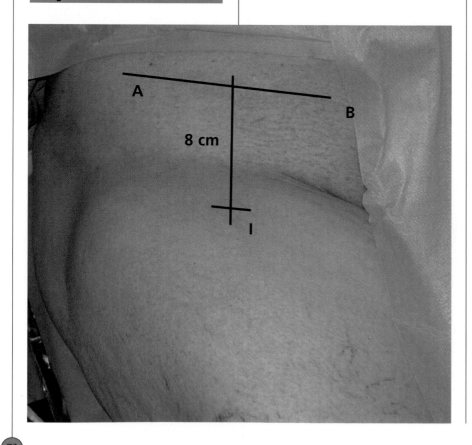

Indications

This approach is indicated for anesthesia and postoperative analgesia for surgery below the knee and may be indicated when other approaches cannot be performed (e.g., in patients with multiple trauma that prevents mobilization of the injured limb or when using more distal approaches).

Continuous anterior sciatic approach. (The arrow in the inset circle indicates the direction of the catheter.)

▼ **Figure 9.8**

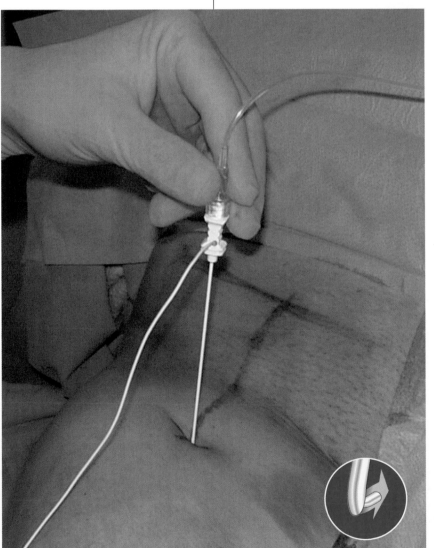

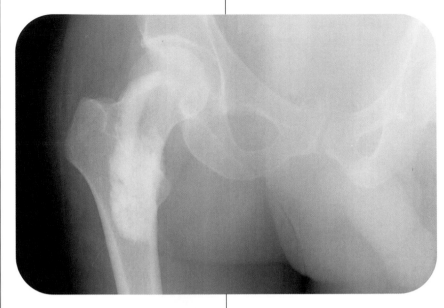

▲ **Figure 9.9**

Radiographic visualization of an anterior sciatic catheter.

Tips

- If bone contact is elicited, the depth at which this occours is marked. The needle is withdrawn to the skin and moved 2 cm medially, and then reintroduced perpendicularly. The sciatic nerve is usually stimulated 2–4 cm deeper than the depth at which the bone was contacted.
- The placement of a catheter with this approach may be more difficult than with other approaches, and is associated with a slightly higher rate of catheter displacement because of the layer of muscle that the catheter has to pass through (*Figure 9.9*).

■ Continuous high lateral sciatic nerve block

Landmarks

The posterior techniques for sciatic nerve block are rather complex and require that the patient or the limb be moved to perform the block. Thus these techniques are less suitable, especially if the limb to be blocked is very painful. However, the sciatic nerve can be reached using a high lateral approach where it is close to and nearly parallel with the femur once it has entered the thigh.

With the patient lying supine and the operated limb at a neutral position, the needle insertion site is identified and marked on the skin, 3 cm caudal from the greater trochanter and 2 cm posterior to the femur *(Figure 9.10)*.

The site of insertion of the needle should be between the greater trochanter and the ischial tuberosity, and can be palpated by placing a hand under the patient.

Landmarks for the high lateral sciatic nerve block.

  GT: greater trochanter;
  I: insertion site, 3 cm caudally and 2 cm posteriorly to the greater trochanter.

▼ **Figure 9.10**

Technique

After appropriate local skin infiltration with 2 ml lidocaine 1%, a 15 cm 18-gauge insulated Tuohy needle, connected to a nerve stimulator (stimulating current intensity 1–1.5 mA, frequency 2 Hz), is introduced perpendicular to the skin, with the tip oriented cephalad *(Figure 9.11)*. The needle is initially advanced to contact the bone, but then it is slightly retrieved and reinserted with the point directed posteriorly at about 20º.

The needle is then advanced until a sciatic-mediated motor response is

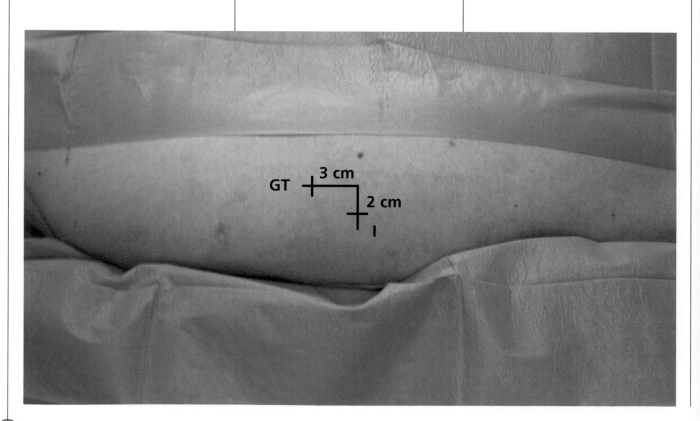

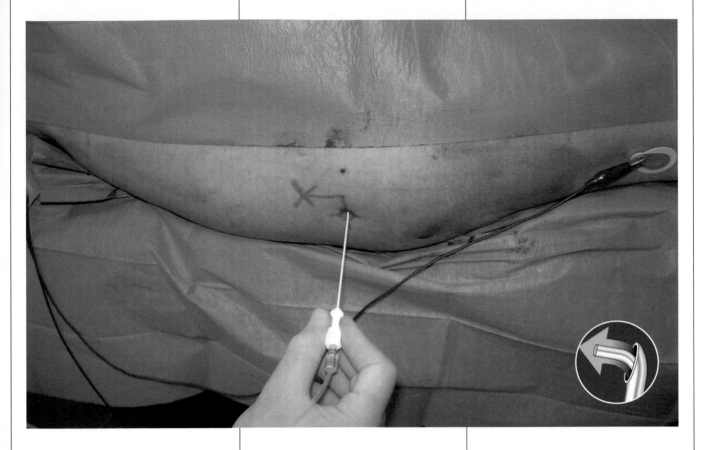

▲ **Figure 9.11**

High lateral continuous sciatic nerve block. The needle is inserted perpendicularly to the skin with the bevel oriented cephalad. (The arrow in the inset circle indicates the direction of the catheter.)

elicited, via stimulation of either the common peroneal nerve (dorsiflexion, eversion of the foot) or the tibial nerve (plantar flexion, inversion of the foot and/or flexion of the toes), usually at a depth of 8–12 cm. The needle position is adjusted until an adequate motor response is observed with a stimulating current ≤0.5 mA, after which 20–30 ml of local anesthetic solution (ropivacaine 0.5–0.75%, or a 1/1 mixture of mepivacaine 1.5% and ropivacaine 0.75%) is injected slowly in 5 ml increments with multiple aspirations for blood.

At this point a 20-gauge epidural catheter is introduced through the Tuohy needle 3–4 cm from the tip, the needle is removed, and the catheter is secured in place.

If the block is used in combination with a femoral nerve block, to minimize the risk of overdosing consideration should be given to the total volume of local anesthetic (no more than 40–50 ml total volume).

A continuous infusion of ropivacaine 0.2% is used postoperatively at an infusion rate of 8–12 ml/h. If a patient-controlled pump is used the infusion rate is set at 5 ml/h with a 2.5 ml bolus and 30 minute lockout period.

Tips

- Placement of a catheter with this approach may be more difficult than with other approaches, but allows easy and simple management of the catheter.
- The incidence and risk of catheter displacement are lower than those observed with the anterior approach.

■ Continuous lateral sciatic nerve block at the popliteal fossa

Landmarks

The classic posterior approach to the sciatic nerve in the popliteal fossa requires the patient to be placed in a prone position, which may be difficult or impossible in some patients (such as trauma and morbidly obese patients). According to the position of the sciatic line, the sciatic nerve can be reached at or above the popliteal fossa, which enables the easy placement of catheters for the continuous nerve block.

The patient is placed in a supine position with the knee slightly flexed by placing a pillow under the leg to make the posterior part of the thigh free. The groove between the lateral border of the vastus lateralis muscle and the tendon of the lateral head of the biceps femoris muscle is palpated and drawn on the skin.

The site of introduction of the needle is located on this groove line 10 cm cephalad to a vertical line drawn from the superior border of the patella (*Figure 9.12*).

Technique

After appropriate local skin infiltration with 2 ml lidocaine 1%, a 10 cm insulated Tuohy needle, connected to a nerve stimulator (stimulating current intensity 1–1.5 mA, frequency 2 Hz), is introduced with the tip oriented cephalad and at 30° posterior to the horizontal plane (*Figure 9.13*).

Initially, a local contraction of either the biceps femoris or vastus lateralis muscle is observed, but within a depth of 4–6 cm these local contractions disappear. Within an additional 1–2 cm a sciatic-mediated motor response is elicited via stimulation of either the common per- oneal nerve (dorsiflexion, eversion of the foot) or the tibial nerve (plantar flexion, inversion of the foot or flexion of the toes).

The needle position is adjusted until an adequate motor response is observed with a stimulating current ≤0.5 mA. Then, after negative aspiration for blood, 20–30 ml of local anesthetic solution (ropivacaine 0.5–0.75%, or a 1/1 mixture of mepivacaine 1.5% and ropivacaine 0.75%) is injected slowly in 5 ml increments with multiple aspirations for blood.

At this point a 20-gauge epidural catheter is introduced through the Tuohy needle 3–4 cm beyond the tip in a cranial direction, after which the needle is removed and the catheter secured in place (*Figure 9.14*).

If the block is used in combination with a femoral nerve block, to minimize the risk of overdosing consideration should be given to the total volume of local anesthetic (no more than 40–50 ml total volume).

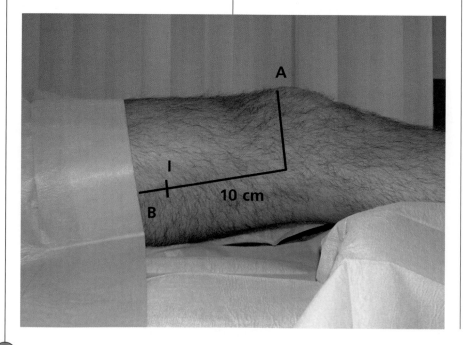

Landmarks for the lateral popliteal sciatic nerve block.

    A: superior border of the patella;
    B: groove between the quadriceps and biceps muscles;
    I: insertion site, 10 cm cranially to the superior border of the patella on the intermuscular groove.

◀ **Figure 9.12**

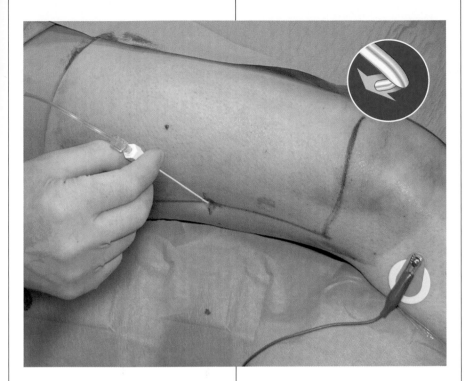

Lateral popliteal sciatic nerve block. (The arrow in the inset circle indicates the direction of the catheter.)

Radiographic visualization of a lateral popliteal sciatic catheter.

A continuous infusion of ropivacaine 0.2% is used postoperatively at an infusion rate of 8–12 ml/h. If a patient-controlled pump is used, the infusion rate is set at 5 ml/h with a 2.5 ml bolus and 30 minute lockout period.

Indications

Continuous lateral sciatic nerve block is indicated with a saphenous or femoral nerve block for anesthesia involving the leg, ankle, and/or foot, and for postoperative pain control, including for ambulatory indications.

Tips

- This approach is very useful in trauma patients, where patient mobilization required by other posterior approaches is difficult and painful for the patient.
- If the sciatic nerve stimulation is not achieved at a depth of 6–7 cm, the needle is withdrawn and reinserted through the same skin puncture, increasing the angle with the skin by 5°, and the maneuvers are repeated until a successful elicitation of the sciatic nerve motor response.

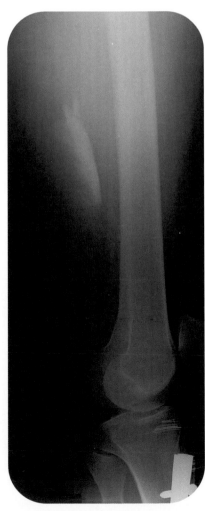

■ Continuous posterior sciatic nerve block at the popliteal fossa

Landmarks

The popliteal fossa is a triangle defined by the tendon of the biceps femoris muscle laterally, the semi-tendinous and semimembranous muscles medially, and the gastrocnemius muscles caudally. At the lower third part of the popliteal fossa, the sciatic nerve is proximal to the popliteal artery and vein.

The tibial and common peroneal nerves are medial to the tendon of the biceps femoris 2–6 cm beneath the skin *(Figure 9.15)*.

The patient is placed in a prone position. The introduction site for the needle is 9 cm from the popliteal crease and 1 cm lateral to the midline of the triangle of the popliteal fossa *(Figure 9.16)*.

▼ **Figure 9.15**

Anatomy of the popliteal fossa.

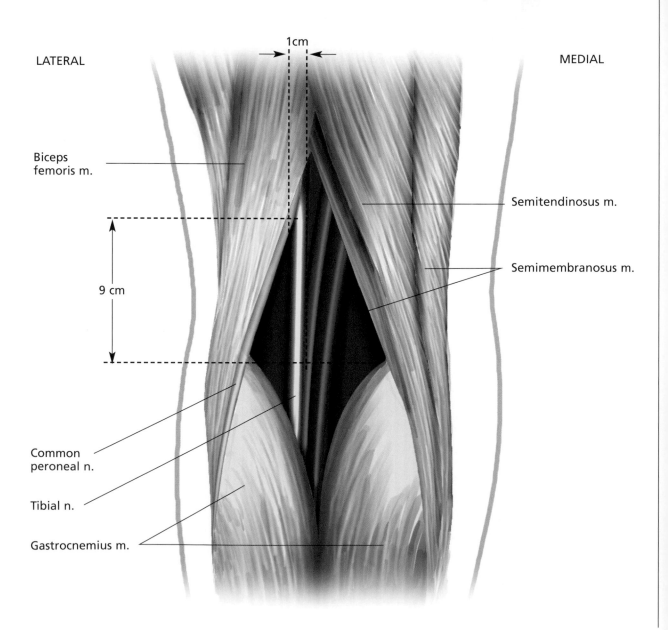

LATERAL

1cm

MEDIAL

Biceps femoris m.

Semitendinosus m.

Semimembranosus m.

9 cm

Common peroneal n.

Tibial n.

Gastrocnemius m.

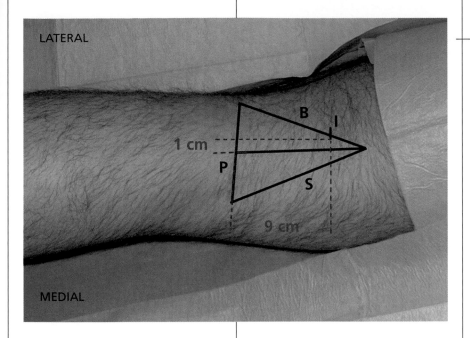

LATERAL

1 cm

P

B

I

S

9 cm

MEDIAL

▲ **Figure 9.16**

Landmarks for the posterior popliteal sciatic nerve block.
- *S: semitendinosus and semimembranosus muscles;*
- *B: biceps muscle;*
- *P: popliteal crease;*
- *I: insertion site, 9 cm from the popliteal crease and 1 cm lateral to the midline.*

Posterior popliteal continuous sciatic nerve block. (The arrow in the inset circle indicates the direction of the catheter.)

▼ **Figure 9.17**

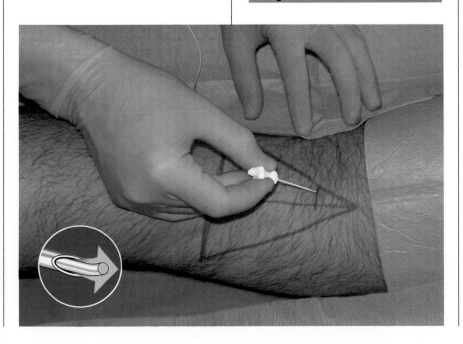

Technique

After appropriate local skin infiltration with 2 ml lidocaine 1%, a 5–10 cm insulated Tuohy needle, connected to a nerve stimulator (stimulating current 1–1.5 mA intensity, frequency 2 Hz), is introduced with the tip oriented cephalad at 45–60° to the skin to facilitate catheter introduction *(Figure 9.17)*. The stimulating needle is advanced until a sciatic-mediated motor response is elicited via stimulation of either the common peroneal nerve (dorsiflexion, eversion of the foot) or the tibial nerve (plantar flexion, inversion of the foot or flexion of the toes).

The needle position is adjusted until an adequate motor response is observed with a stimulating current ≤0.5 mA. Then, after negative blood aspiration, 20–30 ml of local anesthetic solution (ropivacaine 0.5–0.75%, or a 1/1 mixture of mepivacaine 1.5% and ropivacaine 0.75%) is injected slowly in 5 ml increments with multiple aspirations for blood.

At this point, a 20-gauge epidural catheter is introduced through the Tuohy needle 3–4 cm beyond the tip, the needle is removed, and the catheter is secured to the skin.

If the block is used in combination with a femoral nerve block, to minimize the risk of overdosing consideration should be given to the total volume of local anesthetic (no more than 40–50 ml total volume).

A continuous infusion of ropivacaine 0.2% is used postoperatively at an infusion rate of 8–12 ml/h. If a patient-controlled pump is used, the infusion rate is set at 5 ml/h with a 2.5 ml bolus and 30 minute lockout period.

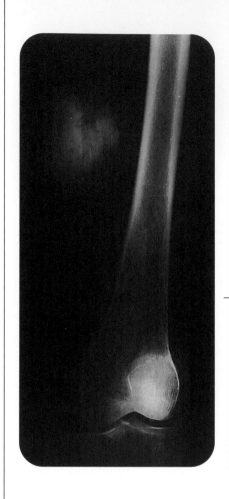

◀ **Figure 9.18**

Radiographic visualization of 5 ml of dye solution injected through a posterior sciatic catheter.

Indications

Continuous posterior popliteal sciatic nerve block is indicated in combination with a saphenous or femoral nerve block for anesthesia and postoperative analgesia in surgery involving the leg, ankle, and/or foot.

Tips

- Stimulation of the tibial nerve usually results in greater success than stimulation of the common peroneal nerve.
- Interestingly, the radiographic visualization of a posterior popliteal catheter is similar to that of a lateral popliteal sciatic catheter *(Figure 9.18).*

CONTINUOUS WOUND INFUSIONS

F.K. Enneking, B.M. Ilfeld

Introduction

The concept of continuous wound infiltration for analgesia is not new. The first double-blind trial comparing wound perfusion with local anesthetic versus saline was published in 1986. In their discussion, Levack et al. (1986) cite historical experience with the technique dating back to 1935.

Innovations in pump technology and in local anesthetic development have spawned a greater interest in these techniques as a component of multimodal analgesia. Rawal et al. (1998) published the first experience of utilizing these techniques for at-home analgesia.

Although much research remains to be done, these techniques have rapidly gained acceptance with surgeons and anesthesiologists because of their relative simplicity.

Abdominal surgery

The most commonly studied case is the use of wound catheters following abdominal procedures. Levack et al. (1986) examined the use of a catheter placed between the peritoneum and the muscle layers following a unilateral subcostal incision for elective procedures.

The patients randomly received a bolus of saline or bupivacaine 0.5% every 12 hours after surgery for 3 days. Those who received bupivacaine had an improved forced vital capacity and reduced narcotic requirements. The pain score, as assessed by visual analog score (VAS), was higher in the bupivacaine group prior to reinjection and lower afterward in comparison with the saline group *(Figure 10.1).*

Factors that may have contributed to the success of this trial were the unilateral nature of the incision and the use of a long-acting narcotic, methadone, for break-through pain. The authors recognized the need for either more frequent 'top ups' or continuous perfusion of the wound.

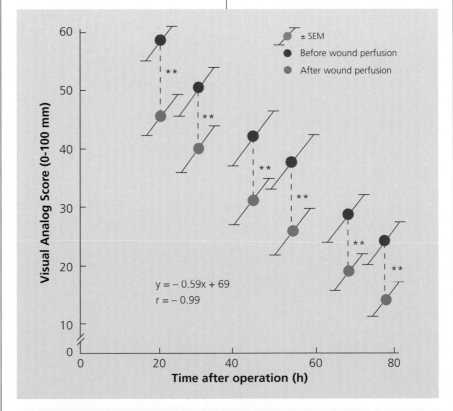

▲ **Figure 10.1**

VAS before and after wound perfusion with bupivacaine (Adapted from Levack et al. 1986, with permission from Oxford University Press).

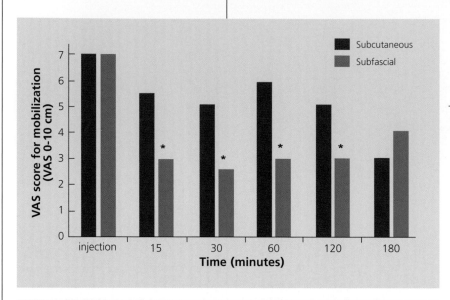

▲ Figure 10.2

Comparison of postoperative VAS score during mobilization with a single 10 ml bolus of lidocaine given to inguinal herniotomy patients either subcutaneously or subfascially (Adapted from Yngaard et al. 1994, with permission from Lippincott, Williams & Wilkins).

More recently, three randomized double-blind studies that examined the use of preperitoneally placed wound catheters following abdominal surgery could not demonstrate a clinically significant difference in pain scores (Gibbs et al. 1988, Kristenson et al. 1999, Fredman et al. 2000). Only one of these studies used continuous infusion of local anesthetic, although at a very low rate (2.5 ml/h); the others utilized intermittent boluses. The lack of efficacy of this technique may be because of an inadequate volume or concentration of the local anesthetic, resulting in its suboptimal dispersion. In addition, preperitoneally placed local anesthetic is not likely to block the visceral pain associated with the surgery.

The location of the catheter may influence the degree of analgesia as well. In patients who underwent inguinal herniotomy, subfascially placed catheters produced a

much longer duration of analgesia than subcutaneously placed ones *(Figure 10.2)*.

Indications

- By itself, an infusion of local anesthetic in the wound is probably not sufficient for analgesia after abdominal surgery, but is most effectively used as a component of multimodal analgesia. In combination with nonsteroidal anti-inflammatory drugs (NSAIDs), cyclooxygenase 2 (COX2) inhibitors and/or oral narcotics it can provide effective analgesia (multimodal approach).
- The catheter should be placed in a subfascial plane and brought out through a site distinct from the incision.
- An initial bolus of 10 ml of local anesthetic into the wound bed should be followed by a continuous infusion of 5–10 ml/h of a long-acting local anesthetic.

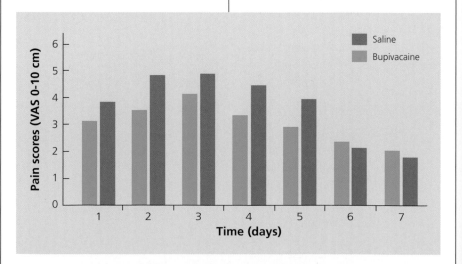

▲ Figure 10.3

Comparison of VAS scores on days 1–7 following subacromial decompression with a 48 hour infusion of bupivacaine versus saline (Adapted from Savoie et al. 2000, with permission from W.B. Saunders).

Table 10.1 Comparison of study group to a matched historical control group following iliac crest harvesting during laminectomy

	Control group	Treated group
PCA morphine usage (mg)		
24 h	90.8 ± 36.4	47.3 ± 25.0[a]
48 h	203.0 ± 48.4	118.4 ± 56.7[a]
Long-term symptoms		
Pain	6/11	2/11[a]
mild	*0*	*2*
moderate–severe	*6*	*0*
Dysesthesia	9/11	4/11[a]
mild	*1*	*4*
moderate–severe	*8*	*0*

PCA, patient-controlled analgesia.
[a]$P < 0.05$ for the difference between control and treated groups.

Adapted from Brull et al. 1992, with permission from Lippincott, Williams & Wilkins.

Orthopedic surgery

Wound catheters have successfully provided analgesia in a multimodal regimen following a number of different orthopedic procedures, including hand surgery, shoulder arthroscopy, and iliac crest bone harvesting. Savoie et al. (2000) found that 48 hours of local anesthetic perfusion of the wound following subacromial decompression led to decreased pain scores for 5 days postoperatively, compared to patients who received saline infusions *(Figure 10.3)*. The control group also used more narcotic and non-narcotic pain medication throughout the study period. Brull et al. (1992) reported improvement in pain scores at 6 months for patients receiving iliac crest wound perfusion compared to historical controls *(Table 10.1)*.

When comparing the direct wound perfusion and continuous peripher-al nerve block techniques, both advantages and disadvantages are found *(Table 10.2)*. Continuous peripheral nerve block provides a more complete blockade of pain from a surgical site. Although low pain scores are recorded with wound perfusion, they are not 0 pain scores, as frequently seen in patients with continuous peripheral nerve blocks. This may be important, particularly during rehabilitation. However, the simplicity of wound perfusion, which requires no special equipment or skill in placement, is a powerful enticement for many patients and surgeons.

The limiting factor for these techniques in orthopedic surgery is the possibility that infection could potentially lead to osteomyelitis. Recently, Axelson et al. (2001) reported three patients with positive catheter tip cultures after shoulder wound perfusion. As orthopedic infections can be devastating, this is a complication that requires routine prophylaxis.

Table 10.2 Comparative advantages and disadvantages from continuous techniques

Continuous peripheral nerve block	Continuous wound perfusion
Visual analog score generally 0–1	Visual analog score generally 3–4
Apparent sensory and motor block	No sensory or motor block
Reinforcement with small patient-controlled bolus	Not studied
Skilled anesthesiologist required for placement	Technically simple to apply
Risk of soft-tissue infection	Risk of wound and bone infection

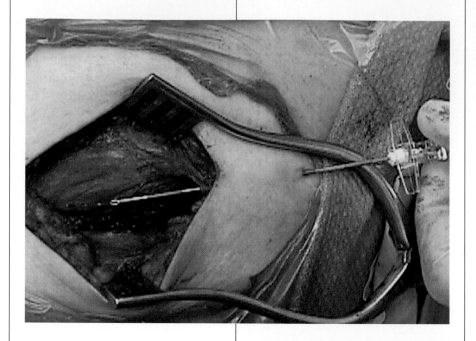

◀ **Figure 10.4**

The catheter is placed in the base of the wound.

The catheter exits at a separate site to the wound. A 10–25 ml bolus of local anesthetic solution is injected followed by continuous infusion at a rate of 4–8 ml/h, based on the size of the wound and the presence of drains.

▼ **Figure 10.5**

Indications

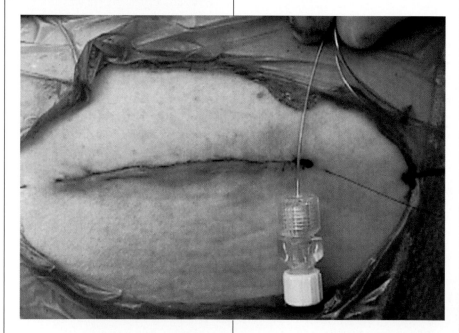

- These techniques are most effective when used in combination with NSAIDs, COX2 inhibitors and oral narcotics as needed. Alone they might not provide effective analgesia.
- Wound catheters should be placed in the base of the wound and the catheter exit at a separate site *(Figures 10.4 and 10.5)*.
- The catheter dose should be 10–25 ml of local anesthetic, based on the size of the wound, to bathe the site with local anesthetic. If a drain is present in the wound, it should be clamped before the catheter is injected.
- An infusion of 2–8 ml/h of a long-acting local anesthetic (such as bupivacaine 0.125–0.25%, ropivacaine 0.2%, or levobupiva-caine 0.125–0.25%) should be initiated. The rate is based on the size of the wound and the presence or absence of a drain in the wound.
- Antibiotic prophylaxis for the duration of catheter placement is strongly suggested for orthopedic patients overall.

CONTINUOUS PERINEURAL INFUSION IN CHILDREN

M. Matuszczak

Introduction

Continuous perineural infusions have been proved to provide effective postoperative pain control in adults (Paul et al. 2001, Sciard et al. 2001), but are still in limited use in children and infants (Rosenblatt 1980, Mezzatesta et al. 1997, Singelyn et al. 1997).

In general, children less than 8 years of age cannot tolerate placement of a block or a perineural catheter while conscious. Therefore, most children who undergo regional anesthesia receive either sedation or a general anesthetic.

With the advent of the nerve stimulator, perineural blocks can be more safely placed under sedation or general anesthesia, and thus can also be used in pediatric patients. This provides the opportunity to place a perineural catheter in children for both prolonged surgery and for postoperative pain management. In older children, depending on sociocultural factors, catheter placement can be carried out without additional sedation, especially when the anesthesiologist is able to gain the child's confidence.

To provide effective postoperative pain management using a perineural catheter, it is essential to inform parents, nurses, and surgeons of the benefits, possible side effects (numbness, motor block), and complications.

■ Indications

The indications for perineural catheter placement and continuous infusion in children are the same as those in adults:

- major surgical procedures on the extremities;
- surgery for congenital malformations of the foot or hand;
- need for long-lasting postoperative analgesia;
- traction of femur fracture;
- sympathectomy for Sudeck's atrophy;
- if parenteral opioids are contraindicated, or for painful physical therapy.

The advantages of continuous perineural infusions have to be compared with those of parenteral or oral medication in terms of quality of analgesia and patient safety. Postoperative pain is frequently poorly managed in children (Rømsing and Walther-Larsen 1996), who receive relatively fewer analgesics than adults (Lloyd-Thomas 1990). Parenteral opioids are the first choice for postoperative pain management and are associated with respiratory depression, sedation, nausea, vomiting, and pruritus. These side effects often limit their administration. Rectal acetaminophen, thought to have an opioid-sparing effect, has proved ineffective for reliable pain relief (Bremerich et al. 2001).

■ Technical considerations

In pediatric practice, the choice of needles depends on the age and weight of the child. Anatomic relationships vary, and bony growth is not the same for long, short, and flat bones.

Variations in the volume of body fluids in compartments and in growth influence the thickness of skin and connective tissues. As a consequence, the distance from the skin to the perineural structures increases unequally with the patient's age.

There are some well-studied relationships between skin-to-nerve distance and the age or weight of the child. These data exist for the following approaches:

- parascalene approach to the brachial plexus [1 cm for a 1-year-old infant to 2 cm for a 16-year-old adolescent (Dalens et al. 1987)];
- posterior approach to the lumbar plexus [2–2.5 cm for a 1-year-old infant to 6 cm for a 16-year-old adolescent; *Figure 11.1* (Dalens et al. 1995)];
- posterior approach to the sciatic nerve [1.5 cm for a 1-year-old infant to 4.5 cm for a 16-year-old adolescent (Dalens et al. 1990)]; and
- posterior approach to the sciatic nerve in the popliteal fossa [1.5 cm for an infant of 5 kg weight to 5 cm for an adolescent of 65 kg weight (Konrad and Jöhr 1998)].

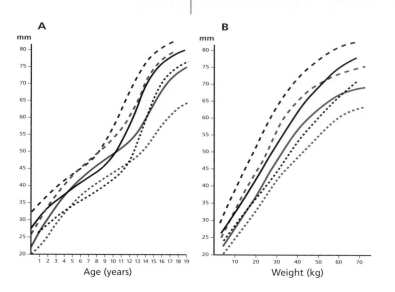

A

mm

80
75
70
65
60
55
50
45
40
35
30
25
20

1 2 3 4 5 6 7 8 9 10 11 12 13 14 15 16 17 18 19
Age (years)

B

mm

80
75
70
65
60
55
50
45
40
35
30
25
20

10   20   30   40   50   60   70
Weight (kg)

▲ **Figure 11.1**

Posterior approach to the lumbar plexus, distance from skin to plexus depending on age (A) and weight (B) for two different approaches: blue, Chayen's approach; black, Winnie's approach. (Adapted from Dalens 1995, with permission from Lippincott, Williams & Wilkins.)

With the above anatomical considerations, the length of the needle to be used should be the shortest that can easily reach the nerve to be blocked, usually 25–50 mm. For the anterior approach to the sciatic nerve, the needle length can be 100 mm.

The types of needles (beveled, external, and internal diameter) and catheters are the same as for adults. Smaller needles and catheters may have a tendency to kink, are difficult to maneuver, and will not allow the blood to reflux. Needle and catheter sizes are, respectively, 18–20 -gauge and 20–22 -gauge. Only insulated needles with a nerve stimulator should be used.

The technique for catheter placement is similar to that used for adults. In addition, after appropriate premedication, the child receives sedation or a light general anesthetic, making sure that a competitive muscle relaxant is not used as this would compromise the use of a nerve stimulator. The child is then positioned as necessary for the approach to be used.

Catheters must be placed under aseptic conditions. The stimulating needle should be introduced carefully because of the short skin-to-nerve distance. As the nerve is localized by electric stimulation and the muscle response is still present at a current of 0.5 mA, a test dose of 1 ml of the chosen local anesthetic solution is injected after negative aspiration for blood. Solutions containing epinephrine (adrenaline) 1:200,000 can be used (Desparmet et al. 1990, Kosek-Longenecker et al. 2000), except in areas with an artery. The effect of the test dose should be assessed for 1 minute before slow injection of the rest of the solution. Aspiration should be repeated during the injection and before all the injections to be carried out later in the procedure. The catheter is introduced through the needle and should be advanced not more than 1–2 cm. The needle is pulled out carefully and the catheter firmly taped to the skin, making sure that it is not kinked. An impor-

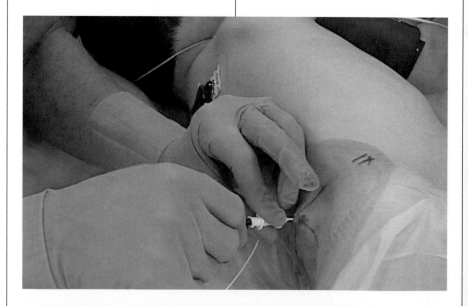

▲ **Figure 11.2**

Dalens' posterior approach to the lumbar plexus.

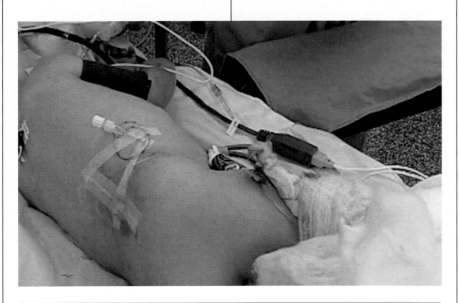

▲ Figure 11.3

Fixation of the catheter to the skin. It is important to ensure the catheter is not pulled out by the child.

tant step during this procedure is to secure the placement of the catheter and ensure that the child cannot pull it out *(Figure 11.3)*. After aspiration, the local anesthetic solution is injected through the catheter. Finally, the catheter is connected to a pump.

Anesthetic solutions

The use of a continuous infusion technique in an infant or child raises questions about the choice, concentration, and rate of infusion of local anesthetics. For the placement of the catheter, any local anesthetic can be used within the pediatric doses. The author's choice is a mixture of equal parts of lidocaine (lignocaine) 1.5% (fast onset) and ropivacaine 0.2% (long lasting) at the recommended doses *(Table 11.1)*. For continuous infusion, ropivacaine 0.2% appears to be the drug of choice in the dose ranges shown in *Table 11.2*.

Like other local anesthetics, the use of ropivacaine is not approved in infants. Nevertheless, local anesthetics are used extensively for neuroaxial blocks, including epidural and caudal blocks (Murat 1995,

Ivani et al. 1998a, 1998b). Ropivacaine 0.2% has been demonstrated to be safe and effective for epidural continuous infusions at rates (Hansen et al. 2000) similar to those used for perineural continuous infusions. Plasma levels have been shown to be below those considered toxic in adults, and no accumulation of ropivacaine after prolonged use occurs in infants older than 3 months (Hansen et al. 2000).

Local distribution is easier in infants, the fat is less dense than in adults and systemic absorption is greater and faster because of the higher cardiac output and regional blood flow. Up to the age of 9 months, the lower level of alpha-1-glycoprotein results in a higher fraction of free local anesthetic, which increases the risk for toxicity. The plasma levels in children are higher than those in adults, and considerable individual variations occur in the peak plasma levels (Murat, 1995).

Table 11.1   Maximum recommended doses

METHOD	Lidocaine		Bupivacaine		Ropivacaine	
Epinephrine (1/200,000)	Yes	No	Yes	No	Yes	No
Epidural (mg/kg)	10.0	7.0	3.0	3.0	3.0	3.0
Plexus block (mg/kg)	6.0	4.0	3.0	2.5	3.0	3.0
Toxic plasma concentration threshold, data from adults (µg/ml)	3.0–7.0		0.3–0.9		1.6–2.0	

Table 11.2   Dosages for continuous infusion

AGE	Bupivacaine 0.25%	Ropivacaine 0.2%	
Newborn*	0.20–0.25	0.2–0.25	mg/kg/h
	0.08–0.1	0.1–0.12	ml/kg/h
Infant	0.4–0.5	0.4–0.5	mg/kg/h
	0.16–0.2	0.2–0.25	ml/kg/h

*30% dose reduction after 48 hours recommended for newborn up to 3 months.

Table 11.3   Children and Infants Postoperative Pain Scale (CHIPPS).
The assessment has to be completed within 15 seconds.
During the postoperative period, values between 0 and 3 indicate a pain-free situation; 4 points or more indicate an analgesic demand with rising urgency.
Repeated observations give more information than a single assessment

Item	Type	Points
Crying	None	0
	Moaning	1
	Screaming	2
Facial expression	Relaxed/smiling	0
	Wry mouth	1
	Grimace (mouth and eyes)	2
Posture of the trunk	Neutral	0
	Variable	1
	Rear up	2
Posture of legs	Neutral, released	0
	Kicking about	1
	Tightened legs	2
Motor restlessness	None	0
	Moderate	1
	Restless	2

Several authors have reported higher levels without any clinical manifestations. However, determination of the local anesthetic plasma concentration in the absence of a relationship between plasma concentrations and the clinical symptoms of toxicity is of limited value in infants. The maximum permissible dose should be considered to be the toxic dose.

■ Pain assessment

Assessment of pain is difficult in adults and even more so in infants and young children. An evaluation supposes verbal communication and visual understanding which may be possible with children who are older than 6 years. At this age a facial expression pain scale or even a numerical pain scale can be used (Dalens 1995). By adolescence, visual analog scales are as reliable as in adults.

For newborns, infants, and young children, a scale for postoperative pain assessment, the Children and Infants Postoperative Pain Scale (CHIPPS), has been tested and validated at the Ruhr-University of Bochum, Germany (Büttner and Finke 2000).

Five observational items are used to identify the need for postoperative analgesics in this age group *(Table 11.3)*. Young children express pain with a range of behaviors to make the signal evident. This scale was validated for postoperative pain and may be less suitable for chronic pain.

Other factors that affect the response to pain must also be considered:

* parents' attitude;
* hospitalization;
* educational and cultural factors; and
* strategies of defense that the child may have developed against painful situations.

Again, the care team should also be involved in this assessment.

Complications

Continuous blockade of peripheral nerves is rarely reported in children and therefore there is little information about specific complications. The most harmful ones are:

* toxicity of local anesthetics;
* trauma to the nerve;
* infections at the site of catheter placement;
* displacement of the catheter;
* incomplete block; and
* allergic reaction to local anesthetic.

High plasma levels of local anesthetic from accidental intravenous injection (connection of the pump to an intravenous line) or an overdose because of erroneous pump settings can lead to central nervous system and cardiovascular toxicity.

The first sign of central nervous toxicity is somnolence and later psychotic manifestations followed by agitation, muscle fasciculation, and finally convulsions with respiratory and cardiovascular depression. However, two case reports in children who accidentally received intravenous injection of ropivacaine did not show any neurological toxicity (Gustorff et al. 1999, Weng et al. 2000). Cardiac toxicity has been reported with bupivacaine and is difficult to correct, but successful resuscitations have been described. The advantage of ropivacaine seems to be its lower cardiac toxicity, as shown in rats (Kohane et al. 1998). Since perineural blocks in children are normally carried out under sedation or general anesthetic, pain as a sign of intraneural injection cannot be expressed. Nevertheless, to the author's knowledge there are no reports of prolonged nerve damage in children (Gioffré et al. 1996, Horlocker and Caplan 2001).

Bacterial contamination can occur during placement of the catheter or during dressing changes. As mentioned above, the catheter should be placed under aseptic conditions and the dressing should be changed on a regular basis. Pressure pain at the insertion site is often the first sign of infection, which should be checked at every visit by the anesthesiologist or pain team.

Displacement of the catheter because of spontaneous movement or during dressing changes is another potential complication. If analgesia is not improved after a bolus of lidocaine 1.5%, it is most likely that the catheter is no longer in the correct position.

The catheter should be withdrawn and parenteral or oral pain treatment relied on. An incomplete block can sometimes be improved by withdrawing the catheter just a few millimeters; however, the child may need supplemental parenteral or oral medication.

Allergic complications are very rare, especially with aminoamides.

Practical considerations

Once the child is on the ward, the care team and, to a lesser extent, the parents have to know about:

- type of catheter;
- reasons for its uses;
- side-effects associated with the technique;
- complications;
- assessment of pain;
- follow up by the anesthesiologist or pain team;
- whom to call if there is any problem;
- records to maintain;
- changing the dressing; and
- how to change the bag and use the pump.

The care team (and parents) must understand that the continuous infusion is part of the pain management and adjuvant medication may be necessary, but to a much lesser degree than without the perineural infusion.

Children sometimes poorly tolerate side effects such as numbness and motor block. They may be ineluctable, but this can often be avoided by decreasing the concentration of local anesthetic solution. The anesthesiologist or pain team in charge should visit the child twice a day, assess the pain, and inform the care team on the ward about all changes in treatment.

The catheter site should be checked every day by pressing on the point of insertion. If there is local pain, the dressing should be changed to look for any sign of infection. If the skin is irritated, the dressing should be changed every day and the catheter withdrawn if any suspicion of infection is present. Under normal conditions, the dressing can be changed every 2–3 days, to avoid an increased risk for displacement.

If the catheter is leaking and still efficient, it can stay in place – some additional layers of gaze may stop the leaking. Depending on the pain, the rate of infusion is continuously decreased and eventually stopped. Then the catheter can be withdrawn or used for bolus injections for painful dressing changes or physical therapy *(Figure 11.4)*. The catheter should only be withdrawn 12–24 hours after the infusion has been stopped, to ensure there is no need for it. The record should be completed, with notes made as to whether the catheter was intact when withdrawn, the skin was normal or not, presence of any paresthesia or motor weakness, and whether the patient and parents were satisfied.

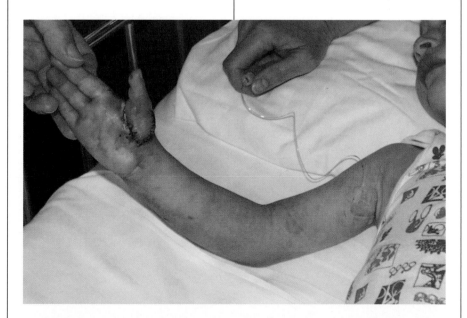

▲ **Figure 11.4**

Axillary plexus catheter in a 2-year-old child, disconnected from the infusion pump 5 days after surgery, and then used for bolus applications for dressing changes twice, before being withdrawn on day 9 after surgery.

■ Medicolegal aspects

Continuous perineural infusion in infants and children is far from being considered as the gold standard for postoperative pain management. Therefore, it is important to choose the best available technique that can be performed safely. The anesthesiologist should be experienced in performing single-shot blocks in children.

A strict protocol for the postoperative follow up on the floor is important (Ivani et al. 2001). The anesthetic procedure should be explained, with its risks, advantages, and disadvantages, to the patient, if old enough, and to the parents. Written informed consent must be obtained from the parents or guardian. An anesthetic record showing vital signs and all details concerning the placement of the catheter and the evaluation of sensory and motor blocks has to be maintained.

References

Abel M, Bahner W, Scholler KL.
Axillary plexus anesthesia in noncooperative patients.
Reg Anaesth, 1983; 6: 58–60.

Auroy Y, Narchi P, Messiah A, et al.
Serious complications related to regional anesthesia.
Anesthesiology, 1997; 87: 479–486.

Axelsson K, Nordenson U, Johanzon E, Gupta A, Rawal N, Lidegran G.
Patient-controlled regional analgesia (PCRA) with ropivacaine after arthroscopic subachromial decompression.
Reg Anath Pain Med, 2001; 26 (Suppl.): 127 (Abstract).

Beck GP.
Anterior approach to sciatic nerve block.
Anesthesiology, 1963; 24: 222–224.

Bremerich D, Neidhart G, Heimann K, Kessler P, Behne M.
Prophylactically-administered rectal acetaminophen does not reduce postoperative opioid requirements in infants and small children undergoing elective cleft palate repair.
Anesth Analg, 2001; 92: 907–912.

Brull SJ, Lieponis JV, Murphy MJ, Garcia R, Silverman DG.
Acute and long term benefits of iliac crest donor site perfusion with local anesthetics.
Anesth Analg, 1992; 74: 145–147.

Büttner W, Finke W.
Analysis of behavioral and physiological parameters for the assessment of postoperative analgesic demand in newborns, infants and young children: a comprehensive report on seven consecutive studies.
Paediatr Anaesth, 2000; 10: 303–318.

Chayen D, Nathan H, Chayen M.
The psoas compartment block.
Anesthesiology, 1976; 45: 95–99.

Chelly JE, Delaunnay L.
A new anterior approach to the sciatic nerve block.
Anesthesiology, 1999; 91: 1655–1660.

Chelly JE.
Peripheral nerve blocks. A color atlas.
Lippincott Williams & Wilkins, 1999.

Dalens B.
Nociception and pain. In: Dalens B (ed). Regional anesthesia in infants, children and adolescents.
Williams & Wilkins, 1995: 35–66.

Dalens B, Vanneuville G, Tanguy A.
A new parascalene approach to the brachial plexus in children: Comparison with supraclavicular approach.
Anesth Analg, 1987; 66: 1264–1271.

Dalens B, Tanguy A, Vanneuville G.
Lumbar plexus block in children: A comparison of two procedures in 50 patients.
Anesth Analg, 1988; 67: 750–758.

Dalens B, Tanguy A, Vanneuville G.
Sciatic nerve block in children: Comparison of the posterior, anterior and lateral approaches in 180 pediatric patients.
Anesth Analg, 1990; 70: 131–137.

Davies MJ, McGlade DP.
One hundred sciatic nerve blocks: A comparison of localisation techniques.
Anaesth Intens Care, 1993; 21: 76–78.

De la Linde CM, Polo A, Lopez-Andrade A.
Continuous axillary plexus block in pediatrics.
Rev Esp Anesthesiol Reanim, 1997; 44: 87–88.

DeJone RH.
Axillary block of the brachial plexus.
Anesthesiology, 1961; 22: 215–225.

Desparmet J, Mateo J, Ecoffey C, Mazoit X.
Efficacy of an epidural test dose in children anesthetized with halothane.
Anesthesiology, 1990; 72: 249–251

Di Benedetto P, Bertini L, Casati A, Borghi B, Albertin A, Fanelli G.
A new posterior approach to the sciatic nerve block. A prospective, randomized comparison with the classic posterior approach.
Anesth Analg, 2001; 93: 1040–4.

Ekatodramis G, Hutter B, Borgeat A.
Efficacy of ropivacaine in continuous axillary plexus block.
Reg Anesth Pain Med, 2000; 25: 664.

Fanelli G, Casati A, Garancini P, Torri G.
Nerve stimulator and multiple injections technique for upper and lower limb blockade: failure rate, patient acceptance and neurologic complications.
Anesth Analg, 1999; 88: 847–852.

Farny J, Drolet P, Girard M.
Anatomy of the posterior approach to the lumbar plexus block.
Can J Anaesth, 1994; 41: 480–485.

Fredman B, Zohar E, Tarabykin A, et al.
Bupivacaine wound instillation via an electronic patient-controlled analgesia device and a double-catheter system does not decrease postoperative pain or opioid requirements after major abdominal surgery.
Anesth Analg, 2001; in press.

Frizelle HP, Moriarty DC.
The 'midhumeral' approach to the brachial plexus.
Anesth Analg, 1998; 86: 447–448.

Gibbs P, Purushotham A, Auld C, Cuschieri RJ.
Continuous wound perfusion with bupivacaine for postoperative wound pain.
Br J Surg, 1988; 75: 923–924.

Gioffré E, Dalens B, Gombert A.
Epidemiology and morbidity of regional anesthesia in children: A one-year prospective survey of the French-Language society of pediatric anesthesiologists.
Anesth Analg, 1996; 83: 904–912.

Gustorff B, Lierz P, Felleiter P, Knocke TH, Hoerauf K, Kress HG.
Ropivacaine and bupivacaine for long-term epidural infusion in a small child.
Br J Anaesth, 1999; 83: 673–674.

Hadzic A, Vloka JD.
A comparison of the posterior versus lateral approaches to the block of the sciatic nerve in the popliteal fossa.
Anesthesiology, 1988; 88: 1480–1486.

Hahn MB, McQuillan PM, Sheplock GJ.
Regional Anesthesia.
Mosby, 1997.

Hansen TG, Ilett KF, Lim SI, Reid C, Hackett LP, Bergesio R.
Pharmacokinetics and clinical efficacy of long-term postoperative epidural ropivacaine infusion in children.
Br J Anaesth, 2000; 85: 347–353.

Horlocker T, Caplan R.
Should regional blockade be performed on anesthetized patients?
ASA Newsletter, 2001; 65: 5–7.

Iskandar H, Rakotondriamihary S, Dixmerias F, Binje B, Maurette P.
Analgesia using continuous axillary block after surgery of severe hand injuries: self administration versus continuous injection.
Ann Fr Anesth Reanim, 1998; 17: 1099–1103.

Ivani G, Mazzarello G, Lampugnani R, De Negri P, Torre M, Lonnquist PA.
Ropivacaine for central blocks in children.
Anaesthesia, 1998a; 53: 74–76.

Ivani G, Lampugnani E, Torre M, et al.
Comparison of ropivacaine with bupivacaine for pediatric caudal block.
Br J Anaesth, 1998b; 81: 247–248.

Ivani G, Conio A, Papurel G, Ciliberto F, Vitale P, Pineschi A.
1,000 consecutive blocks in children's hospital: how to manage them safely.
Reg Anesth Pain Med, 2001; 26: 93–94.

Johnson CM.
Continuous femoral nerve blockade for analgesia in children with femoral fractures.
Anaesth Intens Care, 1994; 22: 281–283.

Kohane DS, Sankar WN, Shubina M, Hu D, Rifai N, Berde CB.
Sciatic nerve blockade in infant, adolescent and adult rats: a comparison of ropivacaine with bupivacaine.
Anesthesiology, 1998; 89: 1199–1208.

Konrad CH, Jöhr M.
Blockade of the sciatic nerve in the popliteal fossa: System for standardization in children.
Anesth Analg, 1998; 87: 1256–1258.

Kosek-Longenecker SA, Marhofer P, Jonas K, Macik T, Urak G, Semsroth M.
Cardiovascular criteria for epidural test dosing in sevoflurane- and halothane-anesthetized children.
Anesth Analg, 2000; 90: 579–583.

Kristensen BB, Christensen DS, Ostergaard M, Skjelsager K, Nielsen D, Mogensen TS.
Lack of postoperative pain relief after hysterectomy using preperitoneally administered bupivacaine.
Reg Anesth Pain Med, 1999; 24: 576–580.

Labat G.
Regional Anaesthesia. Its technique and clinical applications. 2nd edition.
Saunders Publisher, 1924: 45–55.

Lanz E, Theiss D, Jankovic D.
The extent of blockade following various techniques of brachial plexus block.
Anesth Analg, 1983; 62: 55–58.

Levack ID, Holmes JD, Robertson GS.
Abdominal wound perfusion for the relief of postoperative pain.
Br J Anaesth, 1986; 58: 615–619.

Lierz P, Schroegendorfer K, Choi S, Felleiter P, Kress HG.
Continuous blockade of both brachial plexus with ropivacaine in phantom pain: a case report.
Pain, 1998; 78: 135–137.

Lloyd-Thomas AR.
Pain management in pediatric patients.
Br J Anaesth, 1990; 64: 85–104.

Mak PH, Tsui SL, Ip WY, Irwin MG.
Brachial plexus infusion of ropivacaine with patient-controlled supplementation.
Can J Anaesth, 2000; 47: 903–906.

Manriquez R G, Pallares V.
Continuous brachial plexus block for prolonged sympathectomy and control of pain.
Anesth Analg, 1978; 57: 128–130.

Mezzatesta JP, Scott DA, Schweitzer SA, Selander DE.
Continuous axillary brachial plexus block for postoperative pain relief. Intermittent bolus versus continuous infusion.
Reg Anesth, 1997; 22: 357–362.

Morris GF, Lang SA, Dust WN, Van der Wal M.
The parasacral sciatic nerve block.
Reg Anesth, 1997; 22: 223–228.

Morris GF, Lang SA.
Continuous parasacral sciatic nerve block: two case reports.
Reg Anesth, 1997; 22: 469–472.

Murat I.
Pharmacology: Local anesthetics and additives.
In: Dalens B (ed). Regional anesthesia in infants, children and adolescents.
Williams & Wilkins, 1995: 67–104.

Paut O, Sallabery M, Schreiber-Deturmeny E, Remond CH, Bruguerolle B, Camboulives J.
Continuous fascia iliaca compartment block in children: A prospective evaluation of plasma bupivacaine concentrations, pain scores, and side effects.
Anesth Analg, 2001; 92: 1159–1163.

Pham-Dang C, Meunier JF, Poirier P, et al.
A new axillary approach for continuous brachial plexus block.
Anesth Analg, 1995; 81: 686–693.

Raj PP, Parks RI, Watson TD, Jenkins MT.
A new single-position supine approach to sciatic-femoral nerve block.
Anesth Analg, 1975; 54: 489–493.

Rawal N, Axelsson K, Hylander J, et al.
Postoperative patient-controlled local anesthetic administration at home.
Anesth Analg 1998; 86: 86–89.

Rawal N, Fredman B, Zohar E, et al.
Bupivacaine wound instillation via an electronic patient-controlled analgesia device and a double-catheter system does not decrease postoperative pain or opioid requirements after major abdominal surgery.
Anesth Analg, 2000; 92: 189–193.

Ribbers GM, Geurts AC, Rijken RA, Kerkkamp HE.
Axillary brachial plexus blockade for the reflex sympathetic dystrophy syndrome.
Int J Rehabil Res, 1997; 20: 371–380.

Rømsing J, Walther-Larsen S.
Postoperative pain in children: a survey of parents' expectations and perceptions of their children's experiences.
Paediatr Anaesth, 1996; 6: 215–218.

Rosenblatt R, Pepitone-Rockwell F, McKillop MJ.
Continuous axillary analgesia for traumatic hand injury.
Anesthesiology, 1979; 51: 565–566.

Rosenblatt RM.
Continuous femoral anesthesia for lower extremity surgery.
Anesth Analg, 1980; 59: 631–632.

Salonen MH, Haasio J, Bachmann M, Xu M, Rosemberg PH.
Evaluation of efficacy and plasma concentrations of ropivacaine in continuous axillar brachial plexus block: high dose for surgical anesthesia and low dose for postoperative analgesia.
Reg Anesth Pain Med, 2000; 25: 47–51.

Savoie FH, Field LD, Jenkins N, Mallon WJ, Phelps RA.
The pain control infusion pump for postoperative pain control in shoulder surgery.
Arthroscopy, 2000; 16: 339–342.

Sciard D, Matuszczak M, Gebhard R, Greger J, Al-Samsam T, Chelly JE.
Continuous posterior lumbar plexus block for acute postoperative pain control in infants.
Anesthesiology, 2001; 95: 1521–3.

Scott B.
Tecniche di anestesia regionale.
Verducci Editore, 1992; 100–103.

Selander D.
Catheter technique in axillary plexus block. Presentation of a new method.
Acta Anaesthesiol Scand, 1977; 21: 324.

Singelyn FJ, Aye F, Gouvaneur JM.
Continuous popliteal sciatic nerve block: An original technique to provide postoperative analgesia after foot surgery. Anesth Analg, 1997; 84: 383–386.

Tan TS, Watcha MF, Safavi F, McCulloch D, Payne CT, Tuefel A.
Cannulation of the axillary sheath in children. Anesth Analg, 1995; 80: 640–641.

Weng Y, Thong WY, Pajel V, Khalil SN.
Inadvertent administration of intravenous ropivacaine in a child. Paediatr Anaesth, 2000; 10: 563–564.

Tobias JD.
Continuous femoral nerve block to provide analgesia following femur fracture in a paediatric ICU population. Anaesth Intens Care, 1994; 22: 616–618.

Vloka JD, Hadzic A, Kitain E, et al.
Anatomic considerations for sciatic nerve block in the popliteal fossa through the lateral approach. Reg Anesth, 1996; 21: 414–418.

Winnie AP, Ramamurthy S, Durrani Z.
The inguinal paravascular technique of lumbar plexus anesthesia: the 3-in-1 block. Anesth Analg, 1973; 52: 989–996.

Yngaard S, Holst P, Bjerre-Jepson K, Thomsen CB, Struckmann J, Mogensen T.
Subcutaneously versus subfascially administered lidocaine in pain treatment after inguinal herniotomy. Anesth Analg, 1994; 79: 324–327.